**Calculation
of Drug Dosages
a workbook**

Calculation
of Drug Dosages
a workbook

Ruth K. Radcliff, R.N., M.S.NED.

Formerly Assistant Professor of Nursing,
Indiana University School of Nursing,
Indianapolis, Indiana

Sheila J. Ogden, R.N., B.S.N.

Staff Development Associate,
Indiana University Hospitals;
Formerly Resident Lecturer of Nursing,
Indiana University School of Nursing,
Indianapolis, Indiana

FOURTH EDITION
with 105 illustrations

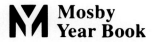
Mosby
Year Book

St. Louis   Baltimore   Boston   Chicago   London   Philadelphia   Sydney   Toronto

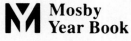
**Mosby
Year Book**
Dedicated to Publishing Excellence

Editor: Nancy L. Coon
Developmental editor: Susan R. Epstein
Editorial assistant: Maria C. Clever
Project manager: Peggy Fagen
Designer: Susan E. Lane

FOURTH EDITION

Previous editions copyrighted 1977, 1980, 1987

Printed in the United States of America

Mosby–Year Book, Inc.
11830 Westline Industrial Drive, St. Louis, Missouri 63146

International Standard Book Number 0-8016-5271-5

C/VH/VH 9 8 7 6 5 4 3

To
Wayne and Mark
for their confidence, reassurance,
and support.

R.K.R.

To
David, John, Amy, and Justin
for their patience, support, and
especially their love.

S.J.O.

PREFACE

This workbook was designed for students in professional and vocational schools of nursing and for nurses returning to practice after being away from the clinical setting. It can be used in the classroom or for individual study. The workbook contains an extensive review of basic mathematics to assist students who have not mastered the subject in previous educational experiences. It can also be used for those who have not attended school for a number of years and feel deficient in mathematics. It may be that a person has not needed mathematics. Today we are very dependent on modern technology; a calculator is used in most activities involving numbers.

To become skilled in mathematics, extensive practice is necessary. Each chapter begins with a pretest for evaluating present skills. Learning objectives are listed so the student will know the goals that must be achieved, the subject matter is introduced, and examples for solving the various types of problems are provided. Work sheets give the student an opportunity to practice solving realistic problems. Two tests evaluate the student's learning. The student skilled in mathematics can easily adapt to applying the skills to solving problems of drug dosages.

The chapter on intravenous flow rates has been enlarged to include intravenous use of heparin, regular insulin therapy, and some critical care titrations.

Three new chapters have been added in this edition of the workbook. "Interpretation of the Physician's Medication Orders" explains what the nurse needs to know concerning prescriptions and orders for medications. "Pediatric Dosages" explains children's dosages and the importance of accuracy in solving problems relating to children's medications. The last chapter discusses "Special Considerations for Administering Medication to the Elderly."

Most problems of drug dosage in this workbook are easily solved using a proportion. The problems concern both child and adult medications, since the method for solving dosage problems is always the same, regardless of the patient's age.

All problems relating to drug dosages presented in this workbook were obtained from physician's order sheets in various hospitals in Indianapolis, Indiana.

We appreciate the physicians, nurses, pharmacists, and representatives of various health care agencies who took time to discuss topics with us. We are grateful to our students, from whom we have learned so much. They have helped us understand the problems students have with basic mathematics as well as with the calculation of drug dosages. We hope this book will provide its readers with a feeling of confidence when working with a variety of mathematical problems.

Ruth K. Radcliff
Sheila J. Ogden

CONTENTS

PART II
Units and Measures for the Calculation of Drug Dosages

PART III
Calculation of drug dosages

INTRODUCTION

The purpose of this book is to provide the student in a school of nursing with a systematic review of mathematics and a simplified method of calculating drug dosages.

To attain the maximal benefit from this workbook, begin at the beginning and work through the book in the order presented. Extensive practice is essential for mastery of mathematics.

Each chapter begins with a pretest to evaluate previous learning. If the grade on the pretest is acceptable (an accepted score is noted at the top of the test), you may continue to the pretest in the next chapter. If the score on the pretest indicates a need for further study, read the introduction to the chapter, study the method of solving the problems, and complete the work sheet. If you have difficulty with a problem, refer to the examples in the introduction.

On completion of the work sheet, refer to the answer sheets in the Appendix to verify that the answers are correct. Rework all the incorrect problems to find the error. It may be necessary to refer again to the examples in the introduction. Take posttest 1, and grade the test. If the grade is acceptable, as indicated at the top of the test, continue to the next chapter. If the grade is less than acceptable, rework all incorrect problems to find the error. Review as necessary before completing posttest 2. Again verify that your answers are correct. At this point, if you have followed the system of study, the grade on the second posttest should be more than acceptable. Follow the same system of study in each of the following chapters.

When all the chapters in the workbook are completed with acceptable scores (between 90% and 100%), you should be proficient in solving problems relating to drug dosage; more importantly, you will have completed the first step toward becoming a safe practitioner of medication administration.

On completion of the materials provided in this workbook, you will have mastered the following mathematical concepts for the accurate performance of computations:

1. Solve problems using fractions, decimals, percents, ratios, and proportions
2. Solve problems involving the apothecaries', metric, and household systems of measurements
3. Solve problems measured in units and milliequivalents
4. Solve problems relating to oral and parenteral dosages
5. Solve problems involving intravenous flow rates
6. Solve problems confirming the correct dosage of pediatric medications

You are now ready to begin Chapter 1.

Review of mathematics

PRETEST

DIRECTIONS: Do the indicated calculations and reduce fractions to lowest terms.

1. $\frac{1}{8} + \frac{2}{3}$

2. $\frac{5}{7} + \frac{4}{9}$

3. $6\frac{3}{5} + 2\frac{3}{4}$

4. $2\frac{1}{2} + 8\frac{1}{6}$

5. $3\frac{13}{20} + 1\frac{3}{10} + 4\frac{4}{5}$

6. $2\frac{5}{16} + 3\frac{1}{4}$

7. $5\frac{6}{11} + 3\frac{1}{2}$

8. $3\frac{2}{3} + 4\frac{2}{9}$

9. $2\frac{5}{8} + 1\frac{5}{24}$

10. $1\frac{3}{4} + 2\frac{3}{8} + 1\frac{5}{6}$

11. $\frac{9}{10} - \frac{3}{5}$

12. $2\frac{1}{4} - 1\frac{3}{8}$

13. $2\frac{2}{3} - 1\frac{4}{5}$

14. $6\frac{1}{8} - 3\frac{1}{2}$

15. $9\frac{1}{2} - 3\frac{5}{13}$

16. $4\frac{5}{6} - 2\frac{1}{8}$

17. $3\frac{3}{4} - 1\frac{11}{12}$

18. $7\frac{1}{2} - 5\frac{7}{10}$

19. $5\frac{1}{4} - 3\frac{15}{16}$

20. $6\frac{1}{2} - 4\frac{2}{3}$

21. $\frac{4}{5} \times \frac{1}{12}$

22. $\frac{3}{8} \times \frac{7}{10}$

23. $1\frac{1}{3} \times 3\frac{3}{4}$

24. $3\frac{2}{7} \times 2\frac{2}{9}$

25. $\frac{5}{8} \times 1\frac{5}{7}$

26. $\frac{1}{1000} \times \frac{1}{10}$

27. $2\frac{4}{9} \times 1\frac{3}{4}$

4

28. $3\frac{7}{15} \times 1\frac{3}{5}$

29. $4\frac{1}{6} \times 2\frac{9}{10}$

30. $1\frac{1}{8} \times 2\frac{4}{7}$

31. $\frac{1}{4} \div \frac{4}{5}$

32. $1\frac{5}{9} \div 2\frac{4}{7}$

33. $2\frac{1}{6} \div 1\frac{5}{8}$

34. $\frac{1}{3} \div \frac{1}{100}$

35. $1\frac{3}{4} \div 2$

36. $\frac{4}{5} / \frac{3}{5}$

37. $\frac{1}{16} / \frac{3}{4}$

38. $\frac{1}{3} / \frac{3}{5}$

39. $2\frac{5}{6} / 1\frac{2}{3}$

40. $4\frac{1}{2} / 2\frac{1}{4}$

Answers on p. 347.

CHAPTER 1
FRACTIONS

Learning objectives ─────────────────────────

On completion of the materials provided in this chapter, you will be able to perform computations accurately by mastering the following mathematical concepts:

1. Changing an improper fraction to a mixed number
2. Changing a mixed number to an improper fraction
3. Changing a fraction to an equivalent fraction with the lowest common denominator
4. Changing a mixed number to an equivalent fraction with the lowest common denominator
5. Adding fractions having the same denominator, unlike denominators, or involving whole numbers and unlike denominators
6. Subtracting fractions having the same denominator, unlike denominators, or involving whole numbers and unlike denominators
7. Multiplying fractions and mixed numbers
8. Dividing fractions and mixed numbers
9. Reducing a complex fraction
10. Reducing a complex fraction involving mixed numbers

A *fraction* indicates the number of equal parts of a whole. An example is ¾, which means three of four equal parts. The *denominator* indicates the number of parts into which a whole has been divided. The denominator is the number below the fraction line. The *numerator* designates the number of parts that you have of a divided whole. It is the number above the fraction line. The line also indicates division to be performed and can be read as "divided by." The example ¾, or three fourths, can therefore be read as "three divided by four." In other words the numerator is "divided by" the denominator. The numerator is the dividend, and the denominator is the divisor.

A fraction can often be expressed in smaller numbers without any change in its real value. This is what is meant by the direction "Reduce to lowest terms." The reduction is accomplished by dividing both numerator and denominator by the same figure.

EXAMPLE: ⁶⁄₈   EXAMPLE: ³⁄₉   EXAMPLE: ⁴⁄₁₀

$$6 \div 2 = 3 \qquad\qquad 3 \div 3 = 1 \qquad\qquad 4 \div 2 = 2$$

$$8 \div 2 = 4 \qquad\qquad 9 \div 3 = 3 \qquad\qquad 10 \div 2 = 5$$

$$\frac{6}{8} = \frac{3}{4} \qquad\qquad \frac{3}{9} = \frac{1}{3} \qquad\qquad \frac{4}{10} = \frac{2}{5}$$

There are several different types of fractions. A *proper fraction* is one which the numerator is smaller than the denominator. A proper fraction is sometimes referred to as a *common or simple fraction.*

EXAMPLES: ⅔, ⅛, 5/12

An *improper fraction* is a fraction whose numerator is larger than or equal to the denominator.

EXAMPLES: 8/7, 6/6, 4/2

A *complex fraction* is one that contains a fraction in its numerator, its denominator, or both.

EXAMPLES: 2⅓/3, 2/½, ¾/⅜

Sometimes a fraction is seen in conjunction with a whole number. This combination is correctly termed a *mixed number.*

EXAMPLES: 2⅜, 4⅓, 6½

Changing an improper fraction to a mixed number

1. Divide the numerator by the denominator.
2. Place any remainder over the denominator and write this proper fraction beside the whole number found in step 1.

EXAMPLE: 5/3

$$1 \text{ remainder } 2 = 1\frac{2}{3}$$
$$3\overline{)5}$$
$$\underline{3}$$
$$2$$

EXAMPLE: 7/2

$$3 \text{ remainder } 1 = 3\frac{1}{2}$$
$$2\overline{)7}$$
$$\underline{6}$$
$$1$$

When an improper fraction is reduced, it will *always* result in a mixed number or in a whole number.

Changing a mixed number to an improper fraction

1. Multiply the denominator of the fraction by the whole number.
2. Add the product to the numerator of the fraction.
3. Place the sum over the denominator.

EXAMPLE: 3¼

$$4 \times 3 = 12$$
$$12 + 1 = 13$$
$$3\frac{1}{4} = \frac{13}{4}$$

EXAMPLE: 1⅜

$$8 \times 1 = 8$$
$$8 + 3 = 11$$
$$1\frac{3}{8} = \frac{11}{8}$$

EXAMPLE: 2 7/10

$$10 \times 2 = 20$$
$$20 + 7 = 27$$
$$2\frac{7}{10} = \frac{27}{10}$$

If fractions are to be added or subtracted, it is necessay for their denominators to be the same. The computations are facilitated when the lowest common denominator is used. The term *lowest common denominator* is defined as the smallest whole number that can be divided evenly by all denominators within the problem.

LOWEST COMMON DENOMINATOR

When trying to determine the lowest common denominator, first observe whether one of the denominators in the problem is evenly divisible by each of the other denominators. If so, this will be the lowest common denominator for the problem.

EXAMPLE: ⅔ and 5/12
You find that 12 is evenly divisible by 3; therefore 12 is the lowest common denominator.

EXAMPLE: ½ and ⅜
You find that 8 is evenly divisible by 2; therefore 8 is the lowest common denominator.

EXAMPLE: 2/7 and 5/14
You find that 14 is evenly divisible by 7; therefore 14 is the lowest common denominator.

Changing a fraction to an equivalent fraction with the lowest common denominator

1. Divide the lowest common denominator by the denominator of the fraction to be changed.
2. Multiply the quotient by the numerator of the fraction to be changed.
3. Place the product over the lowest common denominator.

EXAMPLE: $\frac{2}{3} = \frac{?}{12}$ EXAMPLE: $\frac{1}{2} = \frac{?}{8}$ EXAMPLE: $\frac{2}{7} = \frac{?}{14}$

$12 \div 3 = 4$ $\qquad$ $8 \div 2 = 4$ $\qquad$ $14 \div 7 = 2$

$4 \times 2 = 8$ $\qquad$ $4 \times 1 = 4$ $\qquad$ $2 \times 2 = 4$

$\dfrac{2}{3} = \dfrac{8}{12}$ $\qquad$ $\dfrac{1}{2} = \dfrac{4}{8}$ $\qquad$ $\dfrac{2}{7} = \dfrac{4}{14}$

Changing a mixed number to an equivalent fraction with the lowest common denominator

1. Change the mixed number to an improper fraction.
2. Divide the lowest common denominator by the denominator of the fraction.
3. Multiply the quotient by the numerator of the improper fraction.
4. Place the product over the lowest common denominator.

EXAMPLE: 1¾ and 5/12 $\qquad$ EXAMPLE: 3⅔ and 4/9

$1\dfrac{3}{4} = \dfrac{?}{12}$ $\qquad\qquad$ $3\dfrac{2}{3} = \dfrac{?}{9}$

$4 \times 1 = 4$ $\qquad\qquad\quad$ $3 \times 3 = 9$

$4 + 3 = 7$ $\qquad\qquad\quad$ $9 + 2 = 11$

$\dfrac{7}{4} = \dfrac{?}{12}$ $\qquad\qquad$ $\dfrac{11}{3} = \dfrac{?}{9}$

$12 \div 4 = 3$ $\qquad\qquad$ $9 \div 3 = 3$

$3 \times 7 = 21$ $\qquad\qquad$ $3 \times 11 = 33$

$1\dfrac{3}{4} = \dfrac{21}{12}$ $\qquad\qquad$ $3\dfrac{2}{3} = \dfrac{33}{9}$

If one of the denominators in the problem is not the lowest common denominator for all, you must look further. One suggestion is to multiply two of the denominators together and if possible use that number as the lowest common denominator.

EXAMPLE: 3½ and ⅔

Multiply the two denominators: $2 \times 3 = 6$

$$3\frac{1}{2} = \frac{?}{6} \qquad \frac{2}{3} = \frac{?}{6}$$

$$2 \times 3 = 6 \qquad 6 \div 3 = 2$$

$$6 + 1 = 7 \qquad 2 \times 2 = 4$$

$$\frac{7}{2} = \frac{?}{6} \qquad \frac{2}{3} = \frac{4}{6}$$

$$6 \div 2 = 3$$

$$3 \times 7 = 21$$

$$3\frac{1}{2} = \frac{21}{6}$$

Another method is to multiply one of the denominators by 2, 3, or 4. Determine if the resulting number can be used as a common denominator.

EXAMPLE: ¾ and ⅛ and ⁵⁄₁₂

Multiply the denominator 8 by 3. $8 \times 3 = 24$

$$\frac{3}{4} = \frac{?}{24} \qquad \frac{1}{8} = \frac{?}{24} \qquad \frac{5}{12} = \frac{?}{24}$$

$$24 \div 4 = 6 \qquad 24 \div 8 = 3 \qquad 24 \div 12 = 2$$

$$6 \times 3 = 18 \qquad 3 \times 1 = 3 \qquad 2 \times 5 = 10$$

$$\frac{3}{4} = \frac{18}{24} \qquad \frac{1}{8} = \frac{3}{24} \qquad \frac{5}{12} = \frac{10}{24}$$

ADDITION OF FRACTIONS
Addition of fractions having the same denominator

1. Add the numerators.
2. Place the sum over the common denominator.
3. Reduce to lowest terms.

EXAMPLE: ⅐ + ²⁄₇   EXAMPLE: ⅛ + ⅜

$$\frac{1}{7} + \frac{2}{7} = \qquad\qquad \frac{1}{8} + \frac{3}{8} =$$

$$\frac{1+2}{7} = \qquad\qquad \frac{1+3}{8} =$$

$$\frac{3}{7} \qquad\qquad\qquad \frac{4}{8} = \frac{1}{2}$$

Addition of fractions with unlike denominators

1. Change the fractions to equivalent fractions with the lowest common denominator.
2. Add the numerators.
3. Place the sum over the lowest common denominator.
4. Reduce to lowest terms.

EXAMPLE: $\frac{2}{3} + \frac{1}{5}$

$$\frac{2}{3} + \frac{1}{5} =$$

$$\frac{10}{15} + \frac{3}{15} =$$

$$\frac{10 + 3}{15} =$$

$$\frac{13}{15}$$

EXAMPLE: $\frac{1}{6} + \frac{1}{4} + \frac{1}{3}$

$$\frac{1}{6} + \frac{1}{4} + \frac{1}{3} =$$

$$\frac{2}{12} + \frac{3}{12} + \frac{4}{12} =$$

$$\frac{2 + 3 + 4}{12} =$$

$$\frac{9}{12} = \frac{3}{4}$$

Addition of fractions involving whole numbers and unlike denominators

1. Change the fractions to equivalent fractions with the lowest common denominator.
2. Add the numerators.
3. Place the sum over the lowest common denominator.
4. Reduce to lowest terms.
5. Write the reduced fraction next to the sum of the whole numbers.

EXAMPLE: $1\frac{1}{3} + 2\frac{3}{8}$

$$1\frac{8}{24} + 2\frac{9}{24} =$$

$$\begin{array}{r} 1\frac{8}{24} \\ +2\frac{9}{24} \\ \hline 3\frac{17}{24} \end{array}$$

EXAMPLE: $5\frac{1}{2} + 3\frac{3}{10}$

$$5\frac{5}{10} + 3\frac{3}{10} =$$

$$\begin{array}{r} 5\frac{5}{10} \\ +3\frac{3}{10} \\ \hline 8\frac{8}{10} \end{array} = 8\frac{4}{5}$$

SUBTRACTION OF FRACTIONS

Subtraction of fractions having the same denominators

1. Subtract the numerator of the subtrahend from the numerator of the minuend.
2. Place the difference over the common denominator.
3. Reduce to lowest terms.

EXAMPLE: $\frac{6}{8} - \frac{4}{8}$

$$\frac{6}{8} - \frac{4}{8} =$$

$$\frac{6 - 4}{8} =$$

$$\frac{2}{8} = \frac{1}{4}$$

EXAMPLE: $\frac{7}{12} - \frac{1}{12}$

$$\frac{7}{12} - \frac{1}{12} =$$

$$\frac{7 - 1}{12} =$$

$$\frac{6}{12} = \frac{1}{2}$$

Subtraction of fractions with unlike denominators

1. Change the fractions to equivalent fractions with the lowest common denominator.
2. Subtract the numerator of the subtrahend from that of the minuend.
3. Place the difference over the lowest common denominator.
4. Reduce to lowest terms.

EXAMPLE: ⅔ − ⅙   EXAMPLE: ⁷⁄₁₀ − ⅗

$$\frac{2}{3} - \frac{1}{6} =$$
$$\frac{4}{6} - \frac{1}{6} =$$
$$\frac{4-1}{6} =$$
$$\frac{3}{6} = \frac{1}{2}$$

$$\frac{7}{10} - \frac{3}{5} =$$
$$\frac{7}{10} - \frac{6}{10} =$$
$$\frac{7-6}{10} =$$
$$\frac{1}{10}$$

Subtraction of fractions involving whole numbers and unlike denominators

1. Change the fractions to equivalent fractions with the lowest common denominator.
2. Subtract the numerator of the subtrahend from the minuend, borrowing one from the whole number if necessary.
3. Place the difference over the lowest common denominator.
4. Reduce to lowest terms.
5. Write the reduced fraction next to the difference of the whole numbers.

EXAMPLE: 3⅔ − 1¾   EXAMPLE: 8½ − 3⁴⁄₇

$$3\frac{8}{12} - 1\frac{9}{12} =$$

$$\begin{array}{r} 2\frac{20}{12} \\ -1\frac{9}{12} \\ \hline 1\frac{11}{12} \end{array}$$

$$8\frac{7}{14} - 3\frac{8}{14} =$$

$$\begin{array}{r} 8\frac{7}{14} \\ -3\frac{8}{14} \\ \hline \end{array} = \begin{array}{r} 7\frac{21}{14} \\ -3\frac{8}{14} \\ \hline 4\frac{13}{14} \end{array}$$

MULTIPLICATION OF FRACTIONS

1. Multiply the numerators.
2. Multiply the denominators.
3. Place the product of the numerators over the product of the denominators.
4. Reduce fraction to lowest terms.

EXAMPLE: ⅔ × ⅗   EXAMPLE: ⁴⁄₉ × ⅘

$$\frac{2}{3} \times \frac{3}{5}$$
$$\frac{2 \times 3}{3 \times 5} = \frac{6}{15}$$
$$\frac{6}{15} = \frac{2}{5}$$

$$\frac{4}{9} \times \frac{4}{5}$$
$$\frac{4 \times 4}{9 \times 5} = \frac{16}{45}$$

The process of multiplying fractions may be shortened by cancelling. In other words, numbers common to the numerators and denominators may be divided or cancelled out.

EXAMPLE: ⅔ × ⅗   EXAMPLE: ⁷⁄₂₀ × ⅖ × ³⁄₁₄

$$\frac{2}{\overset{3}{\cancel{3}}} \times \frac{\overset{1}{\cancel{3}}}{5} = \frac{2 \times 1}{1 \times 5} = \frac{2}{5}$$

$$\frac{\overset{1}{\cancel{7}}}{\underset{10}{\cancel{20}}} \times \frac{\overset{1}{\cancel{2}}}{5} \times \frac{3}{\underset{2}{\cancel{14}}} =$$

$$\frac{1 \times 1 \times 3}{10 \times 5 \times 2} = \frac{3}{100}$$

EXAMPLE: ²⁄₆ × ¾

$$\frac{\overset{1}{\cancel{2}}}{\underset{2}{\cancel{6}}} \times \frac{\overset{1}{\cancel{3}}}{\underset{2}{\cancel{4}}} = \frac{1 \times 1}{2 \times 2} = \frac{1}{4}$$

Multiplication of mixed numbers

1. Change each mixed number to an improper fraction.
2. Multiply the numerators.
3. Multiply the denominators.
4. Place the product of the numerators over the product of the denominators.
5. Reduce the fraction to lowest terms.

EXAMPLE: 1½ × 2¼   EXAMPLE: 2 × 3⅚

$$\frac{3}{2} \times \frac{9}{4} =$$

$$\frac{3 \times 9}{2 \times 4} = \frac{27}{8} = 3\frac{3}{8}$$

$$\frac{2}{1} \times \frac{23}{6} =$$

$$\frac{\overset{1}{2}}{1} \times \frac{23}{\underset{3}{\cancel{6}}} =$$

$$\frac{1 \times 23}{1 \times 3} = \frac{23}{3} = 7\frac{2}{3}$$

DIVISION OF FRACTIONS

1. Invert (or turn upside down) the divisor.
2. Multiply the two fractions.
3. Reduce to lowest terms.

EXAMPLE: ⅔ ÷ ⁶⁄₈   EXAMPLE: ¾ ÷ ⁸⁄₉

$$\frac{2}{3} \div \frac{6}{8} =$$

$$\frac{2}{3} \times \frac{8}{6} =$$

$$\frac{\overset{1}{\cancel{2}}}{3} \times \frac{8}{\underset{3}{\cancel{6}}} = \frac{1 \times 8}{3 \times 3} = \frac{8}{9}$$

$$\frac{3}{4} \div \frac{8}{9} =$$

$$\frac{3}{4} \times \frac{9}{8} =$$

$$\frac{3 \times 9}{4 \times 8} = \frac{27}{32}$$

Division of mixed numbers

1. Change each mixed number to an improper fraction.
2. Invert (or turn upside down) the divisor.
3. Multiply the two fractions.
4. Reduce to lowest terms.

EXAMPLE: $1\frac{3}{4} \div 2\frac{1}{8}$ EXAMPLE: $\frac{1}{7} \div 7$

$$\frac{7}{4} \div \frac{17}{8} =$$ $$\frac{1}{7} \div \frac{7}{1} =$$

$$\frac{7}{4} \times \frac{\overset{2}{8}}{\underset{1}{17}} = \frac{14}{17}$$ $$\frac{1}{7} \times \frac{1}{7} = \frac{1}{49}$$

REDUCTION OF A COMPLEX FRACTION

1. Rewrite the complex fraction as a division problem.
2. Invert (or turn upside down) the divisor.
3. Multiply the two fractions.
4. Reduce to lowest terms.

EXAMPLE: $\frac{3}{8}/\frac{1}{4}$ EXAMPLE: $\frac{1}{2}/\frac{2}{7}$

$$\frac{3}{8} \div \frac{1}{4} =$$ $$\frac{1}{2} \div \frac{2}{7} =$$

$$\frac{3}{8} \times \frac{4}{1} =$$ $$\frac{1}{2} \times \frac{7}{2} =$$

$$\frac{3}{8} \times \frac{\overset{1}{4}}{\underset{2}{1}} = \frac{3}{2} = 1\frac{1}{2}$$ $$\frac{1 \times 7}{2 \times 2} = \frac{7}{4} = 1\frac{3}{4}$$

Reduction of a complex fraction with mixed numbers

1. Change the mixed numbers to improper fractions.
2. Rewrite the complex fraction as a division problem.
3. Invert (or turn upside down) the divisor.
4. Multiply the two fractions.
5. Reduce to lowest terms.

EXAMPLE: $2\frac{1}{2}/1\frac{1}{3}$ EXAMPLE: $3\frac{3}{4}/2\frac{1}{6}$

$$2\frac{1}{2} \div 1\frac{1}{3} =$$ $$3\frac{3}{4} \div 2\frac{1}{6} =$$

$$\frac{5}{2} \div \frac{4}{3} =$$ $$\frac{15}{4} \div \frac{13}{6} =$$

$$\frac{5}{2} \times \frac{3}{4} =$$ $$\frac{15}{4} \times \frac{6}{13} =$$

$$\frac{5}{2} \times \frac{3}{4} = \frac{15}{8} = 1\frac{7}{8}$$ $$\frac{15}{\underset{2}{\cancel{4}}} \times \frac{\overset{3}{\cancel{6}}}{13} = \frac{45}{26} = 1\frac{19}{26}$$

14

Study the introductory material. The processes for the calculation of the problems are listed in steps. Memorize the steps for each type of calculation before beginning the work sheet. Complete the following work sheet, which provides for extensive practice in the manipulation of fractions. Check your answers. If you have difficulties, go back and review the steps for that type of calculation. When you feel ready to evaluate your learning, take the first posttest. Check your answers. An acceptable score (number of answers correct) as indicated on the posttest signifies that you are ready for the next chapter. An unacceptable score signifies a need for further study before taking the second posttest.

WORK SHEET

Change the following improper fractions to mixed numbers.

1. $4/3$ **2.** $6/2$ **3.** $9/4$ **4.** $16/5$

5. $17/10$ **6.** $3/2$ **7.** $10/7$ **8.** $13/4$

9. $10/3$ **10.** $19/9$ **11.** $15/10$ **12.** $9/8$

13. $10/6$ **14.** $26/12$ **15.** $19/3$ **16.** $22/7$

17. $35/13$ **18.** $21/6$ **19.** $14/3$ **20.** $11/8$

21. ⁷⁄₂   **22.** ¹¹²⁄₁₀₀   **23.** ³⁷⁄₁₅   **24.** ⁹⁄₆

Change the following mixed numbers to improper fractions.

1. 1½   **2.** 3¾   **3.** 2⅔   **4.** 4⅛

5. 7²⁄₉   **6.** 5³⁄₁₀   **7.** 2⅚   **8.** 1⅗

9. 3⁴⁄₇   **10.** 7⅓   **11.** 4⅞   **12.** 5½

13. 9⅔   **14.** 6⁴⁄₁₁   **15.** 37⁷⁄₁₀₀   **16.** 4³⁄₇

17. 1⅓   **18.** 2⁷⁄₁₀   **19.** 6⅝   **20.** 2³⁄₁₃

18

21. $1\frac{3}{25}$ **22.** $4\frac{1}{4}$ **23.** $5\frac{3}{8}$ **24.** $2\frac{4}{9}$

Add and reduce fractions to lowest terms.

1. $\frac{2}{3} + \frac{5}{6}$ **2.** $\frac{2}{5} + \frac{3}{7}$ **3.** $3\frac{1}{8} + \frac{2}{3}$

4. $1\frac{1}{3} + \frac{5}{9}$ **5.** $2\frac{1}{2} + \frac{3}{4}$ **6.** $\frac{4}{7} + \frac{3}{11}$

7. $2\frac{1}{4} + 3\frac{2}{5}$ **8.** $1\frac{6}{13} + 1\frac{2}{3}$ **9.** $1\frac{1}{16} + 2\frac{3}{8}$

10. $3\frac{3}{5} + 2\frac{7}{10} + 4\frac{1}{2}$ **11.** $2\frac{5}{12} + \frac{5}{6} + 3\frac{1}{4}$ **12.** $4\frac{2}{3} + 2\frac{4}{15}$

13. $1\frac{1}{2} + 3\frac{3}{4} + 2\frac{3}{8}$ **14.** $4\frac{3}{11} + 2\frac{1}{2}$ **15.** $2\frac{2}{3} + 3\frac{7}{9}$

16. $1\frac{3}{10} + 4\frac{2}{5} + \frac{2}{3}$ **17.** $2\frac{1}{4} + \frac{5}{8} + 1\frac{5}{6}$ **18.** $3\frac{3}{5} + 2\frac{7}{8}$

19. $1\frac{2}{3} + 2\frac{1}{6} + 2\frac{4}{5}$ **20.** $\frac{5}{6} + \frac{3}{4}$ **21.** $1\frac{2}{5} + 2\frac{3}{4}$

22. $3\frac{1}{2} + 2\frac{5}{6} + 2\frac{2}{3}$ **23.** $2\frac{4}{9} + 3\frac{5}{7}$ **24.** $5\frac{5}{6} + 2\frac{2}{5}$

Subtract and reduce fractions to lowest terms.

1. $\frac{2}{3} - \frac{3}{7}$ **2.** $\frac{7}{8} - \frac{5}{16}$ **3.** $\frac{9}{16} - \frac{5}{12}$

4. $1\frac{1}{3} - \frac{5}{6}$ **5.** $\frac{7}{10} - \frac{1}{2}$ **6.** $\frac{15}{24} - \frac{7}{16}$

7. $2\frac{17}{20} - 1\frac{3}{4}$ **8.** $3\frac{1}{2} - 2\frac{1}{3}$ **9.** $4\frac{3}{8} - 1\frac{3}{5}$

10. $2\frac{7}{8} - 1\frac{5}{6}$ **11.** $\frac{15}{16} - \frac{1}{4}$ **12.** $4\frac{1}{6} - 2\frac{5}{8}$

13. $5\frac{1}{4} - 3\frac{5}{16}$ **14.** $5\frac{3}{8} - 4\frac{3}{4}$ **15.** $3\frac{1}{4} - 1\frac{11}{12}$

16. $6\frac{1}{2} - 3\frac{7}{8}$ **17.** $3\frac{3}{8} - 2\frac{7}{12}$ **18.** $5\frac{3}{16} - 3\frac{2}{3}$

19. $4\frac{1}{6} - 2\frac{3}{4}$ **20.** $2\frac{3}{8} - 1\frac{1}{12}$ **21.** $3\frac{5}{6} - 2\frac{3}{4}$

22. $5\frac{2}{3} - 3\frac{7}{8}$ **23.** $4\frac{1}{2} - 2\frac{9}{10}$ **24.** $2\frac{5}{16} - 1\frac{3}{8}$

Multiply and reduce fractions to lowest terms.

1. $\frac{1}{3} \times \frac{4}{5}$ **2.** $\frac{5}{12} \times \frac{4}{9}$ **3.** $\frac{7}{8} \times \frac{2}{3}$

4. $\frac{4}{5} \times \frac{5}{7}$ **5.** $6 \times \frac{2}{3}$ **6.** $\frac{3}{8} \times 4$

7. $2\frac{1}{3} \times 3\frac{3}{4}$ **8.** $1\frac{4}{5} \times 3\frac{3}{7}$ **9.** $4\frac{3}{8} \times 2\frac{5}{7}$

10. $2\frac{3}{5} \times 2\frac{3}{10}$ **11.** $1\frac{5}{6} \times 2\frac{4}{5}$ **12.** $2\frac{5}{12} \times 5\frac{1}{4}$

13. $1\frac{3}{5} \times 2\frac{2}{3}$ **14.** $\frac{3}{4} \times 2\frac{3}{8}$ **15.** $2\frac{1}{2} \times 2\frac{1}{4}$

16. $\frac{3}{8} \times \frac{4}{5} \times \frac{2}{3}$ **17.** $1\frac{5}{8} \times 2\frac{3}{4}$ **18.** $\frac{1}{10} \times \frac{3}{100}$

19. $1\frac{9}{10} \times 2\frac{3}{19}$ **20.** $1\frac{3}{4} \times 2\frac{3}{7}$ **21.** $1\frac{5}{8} \times 1\frac{5}{7}$

22. $3\frac{1}{2} \times 1\frac{5}{6}$ **23.** $1\frac{2}{3} \times 2\frac{1}{5}$ **24.** $2\frac{4}{9} \times 1\frac{3}{11}$

Divide and reduce fractions to lowest terms.

1. $1\frac{2}{3} \div 3\frac{1}{2}$ **2.** $2\frac{2}{5} \div 1\frac{1}{3}$ **3.** $5\frac{1}{2} \div 2\frac{1}{2}$

4. $2\frac{1}{8} \div \frac{3}{4}$ **5.** $3\frac{1}{2} \div 2\frac{1}{4}$ **6.** $3\frac{6}{7} \div 1\frac{3}{5}$

7. $4\frac{3}{8} \div 1\frac{3}{4}$ **8.** $3\frac{1}{2} \div 1\frac{6}{7}$ **9.** $7\frac{1}{3} \div 2\frac{3}{5}$

10. $\frac{9}{10} \div \frac{2}{3}$ **11.** $3 \div 1\frac{5}{6}$ **12.** $4\frac{1}{2} \div 2\frac{2}{5}$

13. $2\frac{7}{8} \div 1\frac{2}{3}$ **14.** $6\frac{2}{3} \div 1\frac{7}{10}$ **15.** $5\frac{1}{8} \div 4\frac{2}{5}$

16. ⅞/¼

17. 6½/2⅚

18. 8½/1⁵⁄₇

19. 4⅜/2¾

20. 5½/2⅔

21. 3⅓/1⁷⁄₁₂

22. 3⁷⁄₁₀/2⅘

23. 2⅔/1⁷⁄₉

24. 4½/2³⁄₁₀

Answers on pp. 347–348.

Name _Cristina_____

Date _____

ACCEPTABLE SCORE __36__

YOUR SCORE _____

POSTTEST 1

Directions: Do the indicated calculations and reduce fractions to lowest terms.

1. ⅔ + 4/9

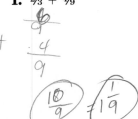

2. ⅜ + ⅓

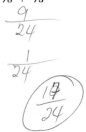

3. 2¾ + 2⅓

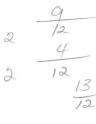

4. 1⁷⁄₁₀ + 2⅗

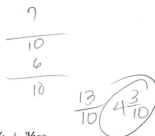

5. 2⅔ + 3/7

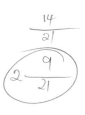

6. 3⁴⁄₂₁ + 1²⁄₇

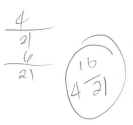

7. ¾ + 3/100

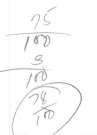

8. ⅝ + 3⅙

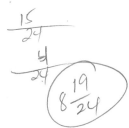

9. 4⅖ + 3¾

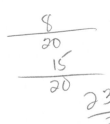

10. 4⅙ + ⅔ + 2¾

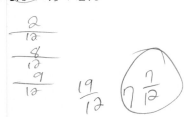

11. 8/9 − ¾

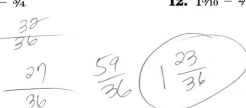

12. 1³⁄₁₀ − ⅖

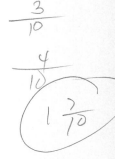

13. 2½ − 1⅔

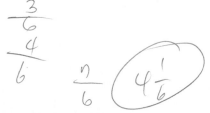

14. 5/7 − ½

15. 5⅑ − 3⅔

25

16. $3\frac{1}{2} - 1\frac{9}{16}$

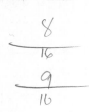

$\frac{8}{16}$

$\frac{9}{16}$

$\frac{17}{16}$ $\boxed{3\frac{1}{16}}$

17. $2\frac{5}{7} - 1\frac{2}{9}$

$\frac{45}{63}$

$\frac{14}{63}$ $\boxed{3\frac{52}{63}}$

18. $3\frac{3}{5} - 2\frac{3}{20}$

$\frac{20}{20}$

$\frac{20}{20}$

19. $9\frac{1}{5} - 3\frac{1}{2}$

20. $2\frac{1}{4} - \frac{7}{9}/\frac{2}{3}$

21. $\frac{3}{4} \times \frac{6}{7}$

22. $3 \times \frac{4}{5}$

$\frac{3}{1} \times \frac{4}{5} = \frac{12}{5}$ $\boxed{2\frac{2}{5}}$

23. $\frac{4}{5} \times \frac{1}{2}$

$\frac{4}{5} \times \frac{1}{2} = \boxed{\frac{4}{10}}$

24. $\frac{2}{9} \times 9$

$\frac{2}{9} \times \frac{9}{1}$ $\frac{18}{9}$ or 2

25. $2\frac{3}{4} \times 1\frac{1}{6}$

$\frac{17}{4} \times \frac{7}{6} = \frac{119}{36}$ $\boxed{3\frac{11}{36}}$

26. $1\frac{1}{4} \times 2\frac{2}{3}$

$\frac{5}{4} \times \frac{8}{3} = \frac{40}{12}$ $\boxed{3\frac{4}{12}}$

27. $10\frac{1}{2} \times 1\frac{2}{5}$

$\frac{21}{2} \times \frac{10}{5} = \frac{210}{10}$ $\boxed{2}$

28. $5\frac{6}{7} \times \frac{3}{5}$

$\frac{41}{7} \times \frac{3}{5} = \frac{123}{35}$ $\boxed{3\frac{18}{35}}$

29. $\frac{1}{4} \times 3\frac{1}{2}$

$\frac{1}{4} \times \frac{7}{2} = \boxed{\frac{7}{8}}$

30. $7\frac{1}{2} \times 5\frac{2}{3}$

$\frac{15}{2} \times \frac{17}{3} = \frac{255}{6}$ $\boxed{2525}$

31. $\frac{2}{3} \div \frac{5}{8}$

$\frac{2}{3} \times \frac{8}{5} = \frac{16}{15}$ $\boxed{1\frac{1}{15}}$

32. $\frac{1}{5} \div \frac{1}{50}$

$\frac{1}{5} \times \frac{50}{1} = \frac{50}{5}$ $\boxed{10}$

33. $\frac{1}{3} \div \frac{1}{2}$

$\frac{1}{3} \times \frac{2}{1} = \boxed{\frac{2}{3}}$

34. ⅚ ÷ ⅔

$$\frac{5}{6} \times \frac{3}{2} = \frac{15}{12} \quad \boxed{1\frac{3}{12}}$$

35. ³⁄₁₀ ÷ 2

$$\frac{3}{10} \times \frac{1}{2} = \frac{3}{20}$$

36. ⁶⁄₇/1⅓

$$\frac{6}{7} \times \frac{3}{4} = \frac{18}{28}$$

37. ⅕/⅓

$$\frac{1}{5} \times \frac{3}{1} = \frac{3}{5}$$

38. 1⅕/⁸⁄₉

$$\frac{6}{5} \times \frac{9}{8} = \frac{54}{40} \quad 1\frac{14}{40}$$

39. ¾/⅙

$$\frac{3}{4} \times \frac{6}{1} = \frac{18}{4} \quad 2\frac{2}{4}$$

40. 3⅛/2¾

$$\frac{25}{8} \times \frac{4}{11} \quad \frac{100}{86} \quad 1\frac{12}{88}$$

Answers on p. 348.

Name _____

Date _____

ACCEPTABLE SCORE ___**36**___

YOUR SCORE _____

POSTTEST 2

DIRECTIONS: Do the indicated calculations and reduce fractions to lowest terms.

1. $\frac{1}{4} + \frac{5}{6}$

2. $2\frac{3}{5} + 1\frac{1}{2}$

3. $\frac{2}{3} + 2\frac{3}{7}$

4. $4\frac{2}{3} + 2\frac{6}{15}$

5. $1\frac{7}{8} + 3\frac{2}{5}$

6. $1\frac{3}{4} + \frac{5}{8} + 2\frac{5}{12}$

7. $10\frac{1}{2} + 1\frac{3}{10}$

8. $4\frac{4}{9} + 2\frac{1}{4}$

9. $1\frac{5}{14} + 2\frac{3}{21}$

10. $2\frac{1}{8} + 1\frac{7}{20}$

11. $\frac{4}{9} - \frac{1}{3}$

12. $2\frac{3}{4} - \frac{7}{8}$

13. $3\frac{1}{2} - 1\frac{2}{3}$

14. $1\frac{5}{7} - \frac{4}{5}$

15. $3\frac{5}{8} - 1\frac{5}{16}$

16. $5\frac{1}{8} - 4\frac{1}{2}$

17. $7\frac{1}{3} - 5\frac{5}{6}$

18. $7\frac{7}{10} - 3\frac{4}{5}$

19. $3\frac{4}{15} - 2\frac{2}{3}$

20. $8\frac{1}{2} - 3\frac{4}{7}$

21. $\frac{2}{7} \times \frac{2}{3}$

22. $3\frac{4}{9} \times 1\frac{4}{5}$

23. $2 \times \frac{2}{3}$

24. $3\frac{1}{2} \times 2\frac{3}{11}$

25. $\frac{5}{6} \times 2\frac{1}{3}$

26. $\frac{1}{100} \times \frac{1}{10}$

27. $1\frac{4}{5} \times 3\frac{7}{11}$

28. $6\frac{3}{4} \times 5\frac{1}{3}$

29. $2\frac{5}{8} \times 1\frac{1}{3}$

30. $3\frac{1}{2} \times 3\frac{3}{14}$

31. $\frac{3}{4} \div \frac{8}{9}$

32. $1\frac{1}{2} \div 1\frac{6}{7}$

33. $2\frac{1}{3} \div \frac{3}{8}$

34. $\frac{1}{7} \div 7$ **35.** $\frac{5}{6} / 1\frac{1}{3}$ **36.** $1\frac{1}{2} / 2\frac{2}{7}$

37. $1\frac{3}{8} / \frac{4}{5}$ **38.** $2\frac{1}{4} / 1\frac{1}{3}$ **39.** $3\frac{3}{4} / 2\frac{1}{6}$

40. $\frac{3}{8} / \frac{3}{9}$

Answers on p. 348.

Name _____

Date _____

ACCEPTABLE SCORE ___63___

YOUR SCORE _____

PRETEST

DIRECTIONS: Write the following numbers in words.

1. 0.04 _____

2. 1.6 _____

3. 16.06734 _____

_____

4. 1.015 _____

_____

5. 0.009 _____

DIRECTIONS: Circle the decimal with the *least value.*

6. 0.2, 0.25, 0.025, 0.02   **7.** 0.4, 0.48, 0.04, 0.004

8. 1.6, 1.64, 1.682, 1.69   **9.** 2.8, 2.82, 2.082, 2.822

10. 0.3, 0.33, 0.003, 0.033

DIRECTIONS: Do the indicated calculations.

11. 184.36 + 2.031 +   **12.** 2.43 + 140.59 +   **13.** 6.8 + 2.986 +
1236.987 + 6.043   839.78 + 0.999   14.7 + 0.89

14. 141.71 + 84.98 +   **15.** 2.5 + 17.292 +   **16.** 1006.48 + 0.008 +
9.98 + 87.63   12.63 + 3.6874   6.2 + 0.179

17. 47.21 + 48.496 + 0.2976 + 54.67

18. 67.276 + 918.9495 + 12.76 + 4.628

19. 5.971 + 63.1 + 8.264 + 7.23

20. 188.646 + 334.72 + 1.3666 + 27.4

21. 2.176 − 1.098

22. 912.13 − 48.68

23. 2.006 − 0.998

24. 836.2 − 76.8

25. 100.3 − 98.6

26. 20.48 − 8.79

27. 0.375 − 0.296

28. 12.6 − 1.654

29. 2.4 − 1.92

30. 34.9 − 26.84

31. 0.63 × 0.09

32. 41.545 × 0.16

33. 0.76 × 0.08

34. 8.053 × 0.024

34

35. 5.25×0.37 **36.** 4.18×0.78 **37.** 44.08×0.67

38. 56.7×3.29 **39.** 8.45×0.08 **40.** 52.9×6.74

41. $0.89 \div 4.32$ **42.** $1.436 \div 0.08$ **43.** $216.48 \div 55$

44. $248 \div 0.008$ **45.** $0.689 \div 62.8$ **46.** $3.59 \div 0.4$

47. $12.54 \div 0.02$ **48.** $13.26 \div 18.9$ **49.** $1.304 \div 0.032$

50. $23 \div 1236$

DIRECTIONS: Change the following decimal fractions to proper fractions.

51. 0.2

52. 0.45

53. 0.008

54. 0.25

55. 0.322

56. 0.27

57. 0.3

58. 0.004

59. 0.34

60. 0.95

DIRECTIONS: Change the following proper fractions to decimal fractions.

61. ⅗

62. ⅔

63. ³⁄₅₀₀

64. ⁷⁄₂₀

65. ¹⁄₁₂

66. ⅝

67. ¹⁄₃₂

68. ⅜

69. ¹⁄₁₂₀

70. ⁴⁄₂₅

Answers on p. 348.

CHAPTER 2
DECIMALS

Learning objectives

On completion of the materials provided in this chapter, you will be able to perform computations accurately by mastering the following mathematical concepts:

1. Reading and writing decimal numbers
2. Determining the value of decimal fractions
3. Adding, subtracting, multiplying, and dividing decimals
4. Rounding decimal fractions to an indicated place value
5. Multiplying and dividing decimals by 10 or a power of 10
6. Multiplying and dividing decimals by 0.1 or a multiple of 0.1
7. Converting a decimal fraction to a proper fraction
8. Converting a proper fraction to a decimal fraction

Decimals are used in the metric system of measurement. The nurse utilizes the metric system in the calculation of drug dosages. Therefore it is essential for the nurse to be able to manipulate decimals easily and accurately.

Each *decimal fraction* consists of a numerator that is expressed in numerals, a decimal point so placed that it designates the value of the denominator, and the denominator, which is understood to be 10 or some power of 10. In writing a decimal fraction, always place a zero to the left of the decimal point so that the decimal point can readily be seen.

Decimal numbers include an integer, a decimal point, and a decimal fraction.

The value of the combined integer and decimal fraction is determined by the placement of the decimal point. Whole numbers are written to the left of the decimal point and decimal fractions to the right. The diagram included here illustrates the place occupied by the numeral that has the value indicated.

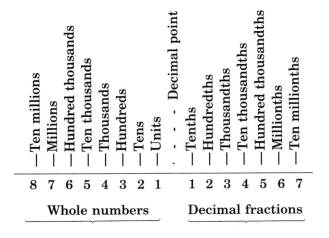

Reading the decimal numbers

The reading of the decimal number is determined by the place value of the integers and decimal fractions.

1. Read the whole number.
2. Read the decimal point as "and."
3. Read the decimal fraction.

EXAMPLES: 0.4   four tenths
0.86   eighty-six hundredths
3.659   three and six hundred fifty-nine thousandths
182.0012   one hundred eighty-two and twelve ten-thousandths
9.47735   nine and forty-seven thousand seven hundred thirty five one hundred-thousandths

Determining the value of the decimal fraction

1. Place the numbers in a vertical column with the decimal points in a vertical line.
2. Add zeroes on the right in the decimal fractions to make columns even.
3. The largest number in a column to the right of the decimal point has the greatest value.
4. If two numbers in a column are of equal value, examine the next column to the right and so on.
5. The smallest number in the column to the right of the decimal point has the least value. If two numbers in the first column are of equal value, examine the second column to the right and so on.

EXAMPLE: Of the following fractions (0.623, 0.841, 0.0096, 0.432), which has the greatest value? The least value?

0.6320

0.8410

0.0096

0.4320

0.841 has the greatest value; 0.0096 has the least value.

Note: In mixed numbers, the values of both the integer and the fraction are considered.

EXAMPLE: Which decimal number (0.4, 0.25, 1.2, 1.002) has the greatest value? The least value?

0.400

0.250

1.200

1.002

1.2 has the greatest value; 0.25 has the least value.

ADDITION AND SUBTRACTION OF DECIMALS

1. Write the numerals in a vertical column with the decimal points in a straight line.
2. Add zeros as needed to complete the columns.
3. Add or subtract each column as indicated by the symbol.
4. Place the decimal point in the sum or difference directly below the decimal points in the column.
5. Place a zero to the left of the decimal point in a decimal fraction.

EXAMPLE: Add: 14.8 + 6.29 + 3.028   EXAMPLE: Subtract: 5.163 − 4.98

$$\begin{array}{r} 14.800 \\ 6.290 \\ +\ \ 3.028 \\ \hline 24.118 \end{array}$$

$$\begin{array}{r} 5.163 \\ -4.980 \\ \hline 0.183 \end{array}$$

MULTIPLICATION OF DECIMALS

1. Place the smaller group of numbers under the larger group of numbers.
2. Multiply.
3. Add the number of places to the right of the decimal point in the multiplicand and the multiplier. The sum determines the placement of the decimal point within the product.
4. Count from right to left the value of the sum and place the decimal point.

EXAMPLE: 8.265 × 4.36   EXAMPLE: 160.41 × 3.527

$$\begin{array}{ll} 8.265 & \text{three place values} \\ 4.36 & \text{two place values} \\ \hline 49590 \\ 24795 \\ 33060 \\ \hline 36.03540 & \text{five place values} \end{array}$$

$$\begin{array}{ll} 160.41 & \text{two place values} \\ 3.527 & \text{three place values} \\ \hline 112287 \\ 32082 \\ 80205 \\ 48123 \\ \hline 565.76607 & \text{five place values} \end{array}$$

Multiplying a decimal by 10 or a power of 10 (100, 1000, 10,000, 100,000)

1. Move the decimal point to the right the same number of places as there are zeros in the multiplier.
2. Zeroes may be added as indicated.

EXAMPLE: 2.64 × 1000 = 2640   EXAMPLE: 0.053 × 100 = 5.3

Multiplying a whole number or decimal by 0.1 or a multiple of 0.1 (0.01, 0.001, 0.0001, or 0.00001)

1. Move the decimal point to the left the same number of spaces as there are numbers to the right of the decimal point in the multiplier.
2. Zeros may be added as indicated.

EXAMPLE: 354.86 × 0.0001 = 0.035486   EXAMPLE: 0.729 × 0.1 = 0.0729

ROUNDING A DECIMAL FRACTION

1. Find the number to the right of the place value desired.
2. If the number is 5, 6, 7, 8, or 9, add one to the number in the place value desired.
3. If the number is 0, 1, 2, 3, or 4, remove all numbers to the right of the desired place value.

EXAMPLE: Round the following decimal fractions to the nearest tenth.

0.168 = 0.2   4.374 = 4.4

EXAMPLE: Round the following decimal fractions to the nearest hundredth.

0.876 = 0.88   2.324 = 2.32

EXAMPLE: Round the following decimal fractions to the nearest thousandth.

3.1326 = 3.133   0.4676 = 0.468

Rounding numbers helps to estimate values, compare values, have more realistic and workable numbers, and to spot errors. Decimal fractions may be rounded to any designated place value. All quotients involving decimal fractions in this book should be extended to thousandths and rounded to the nearest hundredth.

DIVISION OF DECIMALS

1. Place a caret to the right of the last number in the divisor, signifying the movement of the decimal point that will make the divisor a whole number.
2. Count the number of spaces that the decimal point is moved in the divisor.
3. Count to the right an equal number of spaces in the dividend and place a caret to signify the movement of the decimal.
4. Place a decimal point on the quotient line directly above the caret.
5. Divide, extending the decimal fraction three places to the right of the decimal point.
6. Zeroes may be added as indicated to extend the decimal fraction dividend.
7. Round the quotient to the nearest hundredth.

EXAMPLE: 8.326 ÷ 1.062   EXAMPLE: 386 ÷ 719

```
                7.839 or 7.84                      0.536 or 0.54
    1.062ᴀ )8.326ᴀ000                      719)386.000
           7 434                                  359 5
             892 0                                 26 50
             849 6                                 21 57
              42 40                                 4 930
              31 86                                 4 314
              10 540
               9 558
```

Note: the decimal fraction is emphasized by the placement of a zero to the left of the decimal point.

Dividing a decimal by 10 or a multiple of 10 (100, 1000, 10,000, 100,000)

1. Move the decimal point to the left the same number of places as there are zeroes in the divisor.
2. Zeroes may be added as indicated.

EXAMPLE: 358.0 ÷ 100 = 3.58   EXAMPLE: 6.41 ÷ 10 = 0.641

Dividing a whole number or a decimal fraction by 0.1 or a multiple of 0.1 (0.01, 0.001, 0.0001, 0.0001, 0.00001)

1. Move the decimal point to the right as many places as there are numbers in the divisor.
2. Zeroes may be added as indicated.

EXAMPLE: 46.31 ÷ 0.001 = 46,310   EXAMPLE: 5.897 ÷ 0.01 = 589.7

CONVERSION
Converting a decimal fraction to a proper fraction

1. Remove the decimal point and the zero preceding it.
2. The numerals are the numerator.
3. The placement of the decimal point has indicated what the denominator will be.
4. Reduce to lowest terms.

EXAMPLE: 0.86   EXAMPLE: 0.375

$$\frac{86}{100} = \frac{43}{50}$$ $$\frac{375}{1000} = \frac{3}{8}$$

Converting a proper fraction to a decimal fraction

1. Divide the numerator by the denominator.
2. Extend the decimal the desired number of places (often three).
3. Place a zero to the left of the decimal point in a decimal fraction.

EXAMPLE: 4/5   EXAMPLE: 7/8

$$\begin{array}{r} 0.8 \\ 5\overline{)4.0} \\ \underline{4\,0} \end{array}$$ $$\begin{array}{r} 0.875 \\ 8\overline{)7.000} \\ \underline{6\,4} \\ 60 \\ \underline{56} \\ 40 \\ \underline{40} \end{array}$$

$$\frac{4}{5} = 0.8$$ $$7/8 = 0.875$$

Study the introductory material. The processes for the calculation of the problems are listed in steps. Memorize the steps for each calculation before beginning the work sheet. Complete the following work sheet, which provides for extensive practice in the manipulation of decimals. Check your answers. If you have difficulties, go back and review the steps for that type of calculation. When you feel ready to evaluate your learning, take the first posttest. Check your answers. An acceptable sco_ as indicated on the posttest signifies that you are ready for the next chapter. An unacceptable score signifies a need for further study before taking the second posttest.

WORK SHEET

Write the following numbers in words.

1. 0.2 _____

2. 9.68 _____

3. 186.935 _____

_____

4. 0.00008 _____

5. 0.86931 _____

_____

6. 698,437.15 _____

_____

7. 0.0003 _____

8. 12,375.7 _____

_____

9. 6.004 _____

10. 1,968.342 _____

_____

11. 0.02 _____

12. 35.4726 _____

Circle the decimal numbers with the *greatest value.*

13. 0.2, 0.15, 0.1, 0.25   **14.** 0.4, 0.45, 0.04, 0.042   **15.** 0.9, 0.09, 0.95, 0.98

16. 0.5, 0.065, 0.58, 0.68   **17.** 1.8, 1.08, 1.18, 1.468   **18.** 7.4, 7.42, 7.423, 7.44

Circle the decimal numbers with the *least value.*

19. 0.6, 0.66, 0.666, 0.6666   **20.** 0.3, 0.03, 0.003, 0.0003   **21.** 1.2, 1.22, 1.022, 1.0022

22. 0.8, 0.08, 0.868, 0.859   **23.** 0.75, 0.07, 0.007, 0.0075   **24.** 3.015, 3.1, 3.006, 3.02

Add.

1. 1.080 + 31.2 +
   0.065 + 9.41

2. 2.2 + 355.6 +
   8.125 + 6.75

3. 24.684 + 5.3697 +
   8.025 + 2.9

4. 58.7 + 2.5397 +
   4.63 + 822.73

5. 18.95 + 1.903 +
   8.82 + 9.4

6. 5.291 + 17.54 +
   1.32 + 3.7

7. 7.043 + 0.67 +
   13.006 + 1.2

8. 3.096 + 5.892 +
   1.9 + 6.02

9. 1.069 + 2.5 + 1.43 +
   49.034

10. 56.93 + 765.7 +
    64.882 + 7.33

11. 0.3 + 0.874 +
    2.763 + 63.2

12. 9.2 + 2.88 + 4.31 +
    21.004

13. 5.693 + 1.5 + 1.44 +
    14.2

14. 4.6 + 3.291 +
    102.8269 + 0.874

15. 13.5 + 1.023 +
    8.83 + 3.267

16. 1.95 + 14.271 + 5.37 +
    1.8

17. 8.25 + 6.326 +
    6.2 + 20.6521

18. 3.6 + 8.25 +
    2.05 + 24

19. 25.82 + 432.7 +
64.993 + 2.66

20. 0.6 + 0.985 +
1.432 + 52.1

21. 63.65 + 11.73 +
4.005 + 136.895

22. 1.29 + 17.5 +
32.44 + 0.325

23. 3.75 + 0.718 +
136.95 + 0.8

24. 3.64 + 10.49 +
8.65 + 195.27

Subtract.

1. 1321.52 − 63.65

2. 4.745 − 2.896

3. 1.8 − 1.09

4. 42.571 − 9.825

5. 250.7 − 75.896

6. 24.186 − 16.768

7. 1.943 − 0.864

8. 6.33 − 2.186

9. 0.486 − 0.025

10. 1 − 0.012

11. 3.4 − 0.068

12. 8.96 − 2.067

13. 114.3 − 63.625

14. 63 − 0.978

15. 300 − 12.629

16. 0.386 − 0.199

17. 44.892 − 34.943

18. 5.003 − 2.064

19. 1.84 − 0.96

20. 0.013 − 0.004

21. 1036.88 − 117.31

22. 708.6 − 48.86

23. 2.436 − 1.989

24. 47.56 − 29.89

Multiply.

1. 14.376 × 8.025

2. 1.3 × 12.5

3. 29.6 × 5.4

4. 16.4 × 0.4

5. 127 × 4.8

6. 1.69 × 30.8

7. 105×0.25 **8.** 120×5.8 **9.** 9.08×6.18

10. 52.4×0.8 **11.** 7.31×1.6 **12.** 28.9×0.04

13. 3.61×9.33 **14.** 10.2×3.5 **15.** 420×0.08

16. 2.3×45.21 **17.** 325×40.87 **18.** 7.46×54.83

19. 0.64×0.8 **20.** 5.72×7.6 **21.** 6953.64×92.5

22. 1.19×0.127 **23.** 187.5×38.12 **24.** 7.85×3.006

Multiply the following numbers by 10 by moving the decimal point.

1. 0.09   **2.** 0.2   **3.** 0.18

4. 0.3   **5.** 0.625   **6.** 2.33

Multiply the following numbers by 100 by moving the decimal point.

1. 0.023   **2.** 1.5   **3.** 0.004

4. 0.125   **5.** 8.65   **6.** 76.4

Multiply the following numbers by 1000 by moving the decimal point.

1. 0.2   **2.** 0.005   **3.** 0.187

4. 9.65   **5.** 0.46   **6.** 0.489

Multiply the following numbers by 0.1 by moving the decimal point.

1. 30.0   **2.** 0.69   **3.** 1.7

4. 0.95   **5.** 0.138   **6.** 5.67

Multiply the following numbers by 0.01 by moving the decimal point.

1. 0.26   **2.** 90.8   **3.** 5.5

4. 11.2   **5.** 0.875   **6.** 63.3

Multiply the following numbes by 0.001 by moving the decimal point.

1. 56.0   **2.** 12.55   **3.** 126.5

4. 33.3   **5.** 9.684   **6.** 241

Round the following decimal fractions to the nearest tenth.

1. 0.33   **2.** 0.913   **3.** 2.359

4. 0.66   **5.** 58.36   **6.** 8.092

Round the following decimal fractions to the nearest hundredth.

1. 2.555   **2.** 4.275   **3.** 0.284

4. 3.923   **5.** 6.534   **6.** 2.988

Round the following decimal fractions to the nearest thousandth.

1. 27.86314   **2.** 5.9246   **3.** 2.1574

4. 0.8493   **5.** 321.0869   **6.** 455.7682

Divide. Round the quotient to the nearest hundredth.

1. $7.02 \div 6$ **2.** $124.2 \div 0.03$ **3.** $5.46 \div 0.7$

4. $0.145 \div 5$

5. $24 \div 0.06$

6. $67.2 \div 8$

7. $5.44 \div 3.2$

8. $0.986 \div 7.36$

9. $3.7 \div 0.02$

10. $24 \div 1500$

11. $4.6 \div 35.362$

12. $4.13 \div 0.05$

13. $2.22 \div 0.003$

14. $0.412 \div 8$

15. $0.21 \div 0.42$

16. $9.08 \div 2.006$

17. $4.5 \div 3.1$

18. $6.1732 \div 0.355$

19. $63 \div 132.3$

20. $0.56 \div 0.7$

21. $21.25 \div 8.43$

22. $9.2 \div 3.5$ **23.** $75.2 \div 1.6$ **24.** $8.075 \div 0.462$

Divide the following numbers by 10 by moving the decimal point.

1. 6.0   **2.** 0.2   **3.** 9.8

4. 0.05   **5.** 0.375   **6.** 0.99

Divide the following numbers by 100 by moving the decimal point.

1. 0.7   **2.** 8.11   **3.** 700.0

4. 0.19   **5.** 12.0   **6.** 30.2

Divide the following numbers by 1000 by moving the decimal point.

1. 1.8   **2.** 360.0   **3.** 0.25

4. 54.6   **5.** 7.5   **6.** 7140

Divide the following numbers by 0.1 by moving the decimal point.

1. 2.8   **2.** 0.1   **3.** 0.65

4. 0.987   **5.** 15.0   **6.** 8.25

Divide the following numbers by 0.01 by moving the decimal point.

1. 36.0   **2.** 0.16   **3.** 0.48

4. 9.59   **5.** 0.8   **6.** 0.097

Divide the following numbers by 0.001 by moving the decimal point.

1. 6.2   **2.** 839.0   **3.** 5.0

4. 0.86   **5.** 13.8   **6.** 0.0156

Change the following decimal fractions to proper fractions.

1. 0.06   **2.** 0.095   **3.** 0.8   **4.** 0.68

5. 0.125   **6.** 0.74   **7.** 0.0025   **8.** 0.85

9. 0.5   **10.** 0.625   **11.** 0.25   **12.** 0.9

13. 0.004   **14.** 0.12   **15.** 0.055   **16.** 0.875

17. 0.64   **18.** 0.75   **19.** 0.16   **20.** 0.22

21. 0.005   **22.** 0.01   **23.** 0.044   **24.** 0.2

Change the following proper fractions to decimal fractions.

1. ⅛   **2.** ¹¹⁄₂₀   **3.** ⅔   **4.** ⅜

5. ¹⁶⁄₂₅   **6.** ¼   **7.** ¹⁸⁄₇₅   **8.** ⅗

9. 8/200 **10.** 1/3 **11.** 6/7 **12.** 1/12

13. 1/2 **14.** 9/10 **15.** 4/5 **16.** 3/20

17. 7/8 **18.** 13/52 **19.** 3/4 **20.** 17/50

21. 1/200 **22.** 11/125 **23.** 5/6 **24.** 19/20

Answers on pp. 348-350.

Name _____

Date _____

POSTTEST 1

DIRECTIONS: Write the following numbers in words.

1. 42.68593 _____
_____

2. 634.18 _____
_____

3. 0.9 _____

4. 0.003 _____

5. 64.231 _____
_____

DIRECTIONS: Circle the decimal fractions with the *greatest value.*

6. 0.15, 0.25, 0.045, 0.0048

7. 0.1, 0.01, 0.15, 0.015

8. 0.666, 0.068, 0.006, 0.66

9. 0.4, 0.08, 0.6, 0.03

10. 0.525, 5.5, 0.5252, 0.52

DIRECTIONS: Do the indicated calculations.

11. 1.342 + 0.987 + 8.062 + 44.269

12. 2.6 + 4.83 + 0.8 + 0.005

13. 63.9 + 850.6 + 3.8 + 7.743

14. 0.004 + 1.2 + 16.5 + 5.2

15. 0.6 + 0.45 + 2.9 + 4.94

16. 1280.49 + 630.51 + 49.98 + 93.76

17. 11.33 + 9.2 +
     88.75 + 29.16

18. 3.004 + 0.848 +
     0.9 + 1.6

19. 2.875 + 0.75 +
     0.094 + 2.385

20. 1981.62 + 4.876 +
     146.35 + 19.78

21. 93.712 − 4.73

22. 26.521 − 19.384

23. 1 − 0.661

24. 8 − 2.68

25. 2.46 − 1.0068

26. 844.6 − 521.52

27. 1.6 − 0.972

28. 36.892 − 15.942

29. 43.69 − 0.0823

30. 0.9 − 0.689

31. 72.8 × 9.649

32. 1.58 × 0.088

33. 6.25 × 0.875

34. 125.929 × 18.789

35. 360 × 0.45

36. 0.949 × 0.896

37. 26.2 × 1.69

38. 1.5 × 0.39

39. 9846.29 × 93.888

40. 2.6 × 8.42

41. 268.8 ÷ 16

42. 2984 ÷ 0.64

43. 8.89 ÷ 0.006

44. 7.52 ÷ 0.004

45. 462 ÷ 0.009

46. 12.54 ÷ 0.02

47. 56.4 ÷ 40

48. 165.9 ÷ 3.006

49. 0.7 ÷ 0.35

50. 45 ÷ 0.09

DIRECTIONS: Change the following decimal fractions to proper fractions.

51. 0.09   **52.** 0.625   **53.** 0.16   **54.** 0.5

55. 0.0025   **56.** 0.55   **57.** 0.375   **58.** 0.4

59. 0.006   **60.** 0.75

DIRECTIONS: Change the following proper fractions to decimal fractions.

61. 5/7   **62.** 11/50   **63.** 17/20   **64.** 1/100

65. 4/5   **66.** 5/16   **67.** 1/3   **68.** 1/250

69. 1/8   **70.** 3/32   *Answers on p. 350.*

POSTTEST 2

DIRECTIONS: Write the following numbers in words.

1. 0.5 _____

2. 8.2658 _____

_____

3. 4.0002 _____

4. 123.69 _____

_____

5. 2.405 _____

_____

DIRECTIONS: Circle the decimal with the *greatest value.*

6. 0.3, 0.6, 0.8, 0.1

7. 0.25, 0.5, 0.75, 0.9

8. 0.04, 0.45, 0.8, 0.86

9. 0.006, 0.065, 0.65, 0.659

10. 1.202, 1.22, 1.2, 1.222

DIRECTIONS: Do the indicated calculations.

11. 1.2791 + 327.8 +
123.07 + 4.67

12. 101.98 + 4.6 +
9.005 + 14.9987

13. 6.95 + 0.8 +
0.625 + 7.68

14. 19.29 + 3.5 +
5.869 + 4.55

15. 3.75 + 186.857 +
83.3 + 6.988

16. 198.5 + 14.271 +
29.28 + 43.54

17. 823.68 + 459.75 + 723.8 + 4.076

18. 1.5 + 6.3 + 10.46 + 29.465

19. 19.29 + 16.5 + 462.833 + 9.006

20. 322 + 0.95 + 6.45 + 9.6

21. 632.838 − 19.869

22. 32.8 − 4.9

23. 1.572 − 0.985

24. 16.486 − 8.697

25. 6.4 − 3.634

26. 2.6 − 0.087

27. 91.18 − 9.39

28. 11.6 − 7.76

29. 4.819 − 3.734

30. 291.84 − 67.86

31. 14.26 × 2.004

32. 57.6 × 2.9

33. 149.36 × 700

34. 45.5 × 5.45

35. 13.39×2.062 **36.** 56.43×0.018 **37.** 62.41×4.428

38. 12.8×6.5 **39.** 800×3.2 **40.** 27.5×5.89

41. $32.8 \div 0.04$ **42.** $5.9 \div 5.3$ **43.** $0.295 \div 0.059$

44. $537.6 \div 1120$ **45.** $4.89 \div 1.2$ **46.** $124 \div 0.008$

47. $5 \div 2.5$ **48.** $9.6 \div 0.8$ **49.** $0.7 \div 2.3$

50. $5.928 \div 2.4$

DIRECTIONS: Change the following decimal fractions to proper fractions.

51. 0.04 **52.** 0.005 **53.** 0.35 **54.** 0.125

55. 0.9 **56.** 0.85 **57.** 0.003 **58.** 0.8

59. 0.22 **60.** 0.6

DIRECTIONS: Change the following proper fractions to decimal fractions.

61. $^{11}/_{20}$ **62.** $^{1}/_{6}$ **63.** $^{1}/_{400}$ **64.** $^{7}/_{8}$

65. $^{2}/_{5}$ **66.** $^{3}/_{4}$ **67.** $^{1}/_{150}$ **68.** $^{1}/_{2}$

69. $^{1}/_{125}$ **70.** $^{3}/_{16}$ *Answers on pp. 350-351.*

Name _____

Date _____

ACCEPTABLE SCORE ____36____

YOUR SCORE _____

PRETEST

DIRECTIONS: Change the following fractions to percents.

1. 1/60

2. 5/7

3. 1/8

4. 3/10

5. 4/3

DIRECTIONS: Change the following decimals to percents.

6. 0.006

7. 0.35

8. 0.427

9. 3.821

10. 0.7

DIRECTIONS: Change the following percents to proper fractions.

11. 0.5%   **12.** 75%   **13.** 9½%

14. 24.8%   **15.** ⅜%

DIRECTIONS: Change the following percents to decimals.

16. 1⅙%   **17.** 7.5%   **18.** 13³⁄₁₀%

19. ⅘%   **20.** 63%

DIRECTIONS: What percent of

21. 1.60 is 6   **22.** ¾ is ⅛   **23.** 100 is 65

24. 500 is 1   **25.** 4.5 is 1.5   **26.** 37.8 is 4.6

27. $1\frac{4}{9}$ is $\frac{5}{8}$

28. 1000 is 100

29. $3\frac{1}{2}$ is $\frac{1}{4}$

30. 9.7 is $\frac{1}{6}$

DIRECTIONS: What is

31. 3% of 60

32. $\frac{1}{4}$% of 60

33. 4.5% of 57

34. $2\frac{1}{8}$% of 32

35. 4% of 77

36. 9.3% of 46

37. $\frac{3}{7}$% of 14

38. 22% of 88

39. 7.6% of 156

40. 5% of 300

Answers on p. 351.

CHAPTER 3
PERCENTS

Learning objectives ─────────────────────────────

On completion of the materials provided in this chapter, you will be able to perform computations accurately by mastering the following mathematical concepts:

1. Changing a fraction or decimal to a percent
2. Changing a percent to a fraction or decimal
3. Changing a percent containing a fraction to a decimal
4. Finding what percent one number is of another
5. Finding the given percent of a number

A *percent* is a third way of showing a fractional relationship. Fractions, decimals, and percents can all be converted from one form to the others. Conversions of fractions and decimals are discussed in Chapter 2. A percent indicates a value equal to the number of hundredths. Therefore when a percent is written as a fraction, the denominator is *always* 100. The number beside the % sign becomes the numerator.

Changing a fraction to a percent

1. Multiply by 100.
2. Add the percent sign (%).

EXAMPLE: $\frac{2}{5}$

$$\frac{2}{\overset{}{\underset{1}{\cancel{5}}}} \times \frac{\overset{20}{\cancel{100}}}{1} =$$

$$\frac{2 \times 20}{1} = 40\%$$

EXAMPLE: $\frac{3}{10}$

$$\frac{3}{\overset{}{\underset{1}{\cancel{10}}}} \times \frac{\overset{10}{\cancel{100}}}{1} =$$

$$\frac{3 \times 10}{1 \times 1} = 30\%$$

EXAMPLE: $1\frac{1}{4}$

$$\frac{5}{\overset{}{\underset{1}{\cancel{4}}}} \times \frac{\overset{25}{\cancel{100}}}{1} =$$

$$\frac{5 \times 25}{1} = 125\%$$

EXAMPLE: $\frac{1}{3}$

$$\frac{1}{3} \times \frac{100}{1} =$$

$$\frac{1 \times 100}{3 \times 1} = \frac{100}{3} = 33\frac{1}{3}\%$$

Changing a decimal to a percent

1. Multiply by 100 (by moving the decimal point two places to the right).
2. Add the percent sign (%).

EXAMPLE: 0.421   EXAMPLE: 0.98

$0.421 \times 100 = 42.1$ $0.98 \times 100 = 98$

42.1%   98%

EXAMPLE: 0.2   EXAMPLE: 1.1212

$0.2 \times 100 = 20$ $1.1212 \times 100 = 112.12$

20%   112.12%

Changing a percent to a fraction

1. Drop the % sign.
2. Write the remaining number as the fraction's numerator.
3. Write 100 as the denominator. (The denominator will *always* be 100.)
4. Reduce the fraction to lowest terms.

EXAMPLE: 45%   EXAMPLE: 0.3%

$$\frac{45}{100} = \frac{9}{20} \qquad\qquad \frac{0.3}{100} =$$

EXAMPLE: 3½%

$$\frac{3\frac{1}{2}}{100} = \frac{7/2}{100} \qquad\qquad \frac{\frac{3}{10}}{100}$$

$$\frac{7}{2} \div 100 = \qquad\qquad \frac{3}{10} \div \frac{100}{1} =$$

$$\frac{7}{2} \times \frac{1}{100} = \frac{7}{200} \qquad\qquad \frac{3}{10} \times \frac{1}{100} = \frac{3}{1000}$$

Changing a percent to a decimal

1. Drop the % sign.
2. Divide the remaining number by 100 (by moving the decimal point two places to the left).
3. Express the quotient as a decimal.

EXAMPLE: 32%   EXAMPLE: 125%

0.32   1.25

Changing a percent containing a fraction to a decimal

1. Drop the % sign.
2. Change the mixed number to an improper fraction.
3. Divide by 100.
4. Reduce the fraction to lowest terms.
5. Divide the numerator by the denominator, expressing the quotient as a decimal.

EXAMPLE: 12½%   EXAMPLE: 3¾%

$$\frac{25}{2} \div \frac{100}{1} =$$ $$\frac{15}{4} \div \frac{100}{1} =$$

$$\overset{1}{\underset{4}{\frac{\cancel{25}}{2}}} \times \frac{1}{\cancel{100}} = \frac{1}{8} = 0.125$$ $$\overset{3}{\underset{20}{\frac{\cancel{15}}{4}}} \times \frac{1}{\cancel{100}} = \frac{3}{80} = 0.0375$$

```
    0.125                              0.0375
  8)1.000                           80)3.0000
    8                                  2 40
    20                                 600
    16                                 560
    40                                 400
    40                                 400
```

$$12\frac{1}{2}\% = 0.125$$ $$3\frac{3}{4}\% = 0.0375$$

Finding what percent one number is of another

1. Write the number following the word "of" as the denominator of a fraction.
2. Write the other number as the numerator of the fraction.
3. Divide the numerator by the denominator, extending the decimal fraction four places to the right of the decimal point.
4. Multiply by 100.
5. Add the % sign.

EXAMPLE: What percent of 24 is 9?   EXAMPLE: What percent of 5.4 is 1.2?

$$\frac{9}{24} = \frac{3}{8}$$

```
    0.375
  8)3.000
    2 4
    60
    56
    40
    40
```

$$0.375 \times 100 = 37.5$$

$$37.5 + \% \text{ sign} = 37.5\%$$

$$\frac{1.2}{5.4} =$$
```
            0.0222
        5.4)1.2000
            1 08
            120
            108
            120
            108
```

$$0.0222 \times 100 = 2.22$$

$$2.22 + \% \text{ sign} = 2.22\%$$

EXAMPLE: What percent of 2 is ¼?

$$¼/2$$

$$\frac{1}{4} \div 2 =$$

$$\frac{1}{4} \div \frac{2}{1} =$$

$$\frac{1}{4} \times \frac{1}{2} = \frac{1}{8}$$

$$\frac{1}{\underset{2}{8}} \times \frac{\overset{25}{100}}{1} = \frac{25}{2} = 12.5\%$$

EXAMPLE: What percent of 8.7 is 3½?

$$\frac{3\frac{1}{2}}{8.7} = \frac{3.5}{8.7}$$

$$\begin{array}{r} 0.0402 \\ 8.7\overline{)3.5000} \\ \underline{3\ 48} \\ 20 \\ \underline{00} \\ 200 \\ \underline{174} \\ 26 \end{array}$$

$$0.0402 \times 100 = 4.02$$

$$4.02 + \%\ \text{sign} = 4.02\%$$

Finding the given percent of a number

1. Write the percent as a decimal number.
2. Multiply by the other number.

EXAMPLE: What is 40% of 180?

$$\frac{40}{100} = 100\overline{)40.0} \quad \begin{array}{r} 0.4 \\ \underline{40\ 0} \end{array}$$

$$\begin{array}{r} 180 \\ \times\ 0.4 \\ \hline 72.0 \end{array}$$

$$40\% \text{ of } 180 = 72$$

EXAMPLE: What is 3⁄10% of 52?

$$\frac{\frac{3}{10}}{100} = \frac{3}{10} \div \frac{100}{1} =$$

$$\frac{3}{10} \times \frac{1}{100} = \frac{3}{1000}$$

$$\frac{3}{1000} = 0.003$$

$$\begin{array}{r} 0.003 \\ \times\ 52 \\ \hline 0\ 006 \\ 00\ 15 \\ \hline 00.156 \end{array}$$

$$3⁄10\% \text{ of } 52 = 0.156$$

Study the introductory material. The processes for the calculation of the problems are listed in steps. Memorize the steps for each calculation before beginning the work sheet. Complete the following work sheet, which provides for extensive practice in the manipulation of percents. Check your answers. If you have any difficulty, go back and review the steps for that type of calculation. When you feel ready to evaluate your learning, take the first posttest. Check your answers. An acceptable score as indicated on the posttest signifies that you are ready for the next chapter. An unacceptable score signifies a need for further study before taking the second posttest.

WORK SHEET

Change each of the following proper fractions to a percent.

1. ¾

2. ½

3. ⅜

4. ⅘

5. 8/25

6. 3/1000

7. 7/200

8. ⅔

9. 5/12

10. 7/30

11. 9/400

12. 27/32

13. 3/20

14. 12/17

15. 5/22

16. 9/150

17. 11/16

18. 3/14

19. 8/21

20. ⅚

21. 75/10,000   **22.** 2/15   **23.** 4/9   **24.** 7/8

Change each of the following decimals to a percent.

1. 0.402   **2.** 0.0367   **3.** 4.31   **4.** 0.163

5. 6.22   **6.** 0.98   **7.** 0.3276   **8.** 0.3

9. 1.3397   **10.** 0.145   **11.** 0.2824   **12.** 0.67

13. 0.7   **14.** 0.62240   **15.** 0.42   **16.** 0.6337

17. 6.2   **18.** 0.159   **19.** 2.9014   **20.** 0.673

21. 0.405   **22.** 0.3712   **23.** 7.234   **24.** 2.2

Change each of the following percents to a mixed number or a proper fraction.

1. 3.5%   **2.** ¾%   **3.** 40.6%   **4.** 0.125%

5. 10%   **6.** ⅔%   **7.** ⅙%   **8.** 0.35%

9. 45%   **10.** 20.2%   **11.** ⅝%   **12.** 4½%

13. 12%   **14.** 0.25%   **15.** 2⅜%   **16.** 58%

17. 8%   **18.** 6¼%   **19.** 2.1%   **20.** 0.15%

21. 0.5%   **22.** 32.4%   **23.** 66⅔%   **24.** 1.8%

Change each of the following percents to a decimal.

1. 37.5%   **2.** 3%   **3.** 17⁄10%   **4.** 6¾%

5. 0.42%   **6.** ¼%   **7.** 40%   **8.** 1.35%

9. 2½%   **10.** ⅜%   **11.** 5%   **12.** 80%

13. 0.23%   **14.** 72.6%   **15.** 16%   **16.** 30.64%

17. 2.93%   **18.** 5⁄16%   **19.** 87.5%   **20.** ½%

21. 5¾%   **22.** 0.98%   **23.** 6⁹⁄₁₀%   **24.** ⁷⁄₁₂%

What percent of

1. 40 is 22   **2.** 72 is 12   **3.** 80 is 6.3   **4.** 60 is 30

5. 150 is 70   **6.** 500 is 420   **7.** 22 is 5.4   **8.** 50 is 100

9. 144 is 8.2   **10.** 200 is 4   **11.** 500 is 60   **12.** 20 is 1

13. 24 is 3.6   **14.** 325 is 75   **15.** 163 is 121   **16.** 275 is 55

17. 1000 is 100   **18.** 750 is 35.6   **19.** 76 is 8.2   **20.** 800 is 360

21. 25 is ¼   **22.** 250 is 5.2   **23.** 10 is ⅜   **24.** 35 is 7

What is

1. 25% of 478   **2.** 10% of 34   **3.** 2.8% of 510

4. 75% of 845   **5.** ½% of 28   **6.** 0.25% of 650

7. 85% of 36.2   **8.** 33⅓% of 3000   **9.** 3.5% of 57

10. 1% of 400   **11.** 12% of 96   **12.** ⅕% of 65

13. 2¼% of 26   **14.** ⅜% of 32   **15.** 44.8% of 294

16. 62% of 871

17. ¼% of 68

18. 41% of 27

19. 72% of 234

20. ⅓% of 20

21. 8.4% of 128

22. 150% of 70

23. ³⁄₁₆% of 54

24. 6% of 84.78

Answers on pp. 351-352.

Name _____

Date _____

ACCEPTABLE SCORE ___**36**___

YOUR SCORE _____

POSTTEST 1

DIRECTIONS: Change the following fractions to percents.

1. $\frac{4}{9}$

2. $\frac{7}{8}$

3. $\frac{11}{20}$

4. $\frac{8}{3}$

5. $\frac{3}{1000}$

DIRECTIONS: Change the following decimals to percents.

6. 0.256

7. 33.3

8. 0.004

9. 1.678

10. 0.9

DIRECTIONS: Change the following percents to proper fractions.

11. 60%   **12.** 85%   **13.** 0.3%

14. ¼%   **15.** 3½%

DIRECTIONS: Change the following percents to decimals.

16. 86.3%   **17.** 4⅝%   **18.** 29.45%

19. ⅞%   **20.** 0.36%

DIRECTIONS: What percent of

21. 70 is 7   **22.** 24 is 1.2   **23.** 300 is 1

24. 66⅔ is 8   **25.** 3.5 is 1.5   **26.** 2.5 is 0.5

27. ¾ is ⅜

28. 160 is 12

29. 65 is 5.5

30. 250 is 20

DIRECTIONS: WHAT IS

31. 65% of 800

32. 90% of 40

33. ⅛% of 72

34. 8.5% of 2000

35. 2¼% of 75

36. 4½% of 940

37. 65% of 450

38. ¼% of 60

39. 4.3% of 56

40. 0.52% of 88

Answers on p. 352.

Name _____

Date _____

ACCEPTABLE SCORE ___36___

YOUR SCORE _____

POSTTEST 2

DIRECTIONS: Change the following fractions to percents.

1. $\frac{1}{8}$

2. $\frac{2}{5}$

3. $\frac{1}{6}$

4. $\frac{19}{20}$

5. $\frac{11}{9}$

DIRECTIONS: Change the following decimals to percents.

6. 0.065

7. 0.005

8. 4.346

9. 0.57

10. 0.2

DIRECTIONS: Change the following percents to proper fractions.

11. 0.3% **12.** 16½% **13.** ⅗%

14. 1.75% **15.** 0.25%

DIRECTIONS: Change the following percents to decimals.

16. 0.4% **17.** 3¾% **18.** 7%

19. 5.55% **20.** 65%

DIRECTIONS: What percent of

21. 5.4 is 1.2 **22.** ¼ is ⅛ **23.** 250 is 6

24. 40 is 32 **25.** 160 is 12 **26.** 500 is 50

27. 5¾ is 2⅜   **28.** 120 is 15   **29.** 8.7 is 3½

30. 9⁄16 is 5⁄7

Directions: What is

31. 35% of 650   **32.** ¼% of 116   **33.** 4½% of 940

34. 11% of 88   **35.** 16% of 90   **36.** 7.5% of 261

37. 45% of 24.27   **38.** ⅞% of 64   **39.** 3⁄10% of 52

40. 82.4% of 118   *Answers on p. 352.*

Name _____

Date _____

ACCEPTABLE SCORE ___27___

YOUR SCORE _____

PRETEST

DIRECTIONS: Convert to equivalents.

	Ratio	**Fraction**	**Decimal**	**Percent**
1	17:51			
2			0.715	
3		8/20		
4				12½%
5	21:420			
6		5/32		
7			0.286	
8				71³/₇%
9				16¼%
10			0.462	

Answers on p. 352.

CHAPTER 4
RATIOS

Learning objectives

On the completion of the materials provided in this chapter, you will be able to perform computations by mastering the following mathematical concepts:

1. Changing a proper fraction, decimal fraction, and percent to a ratio reduced to lowest terms.
2. Changing a ratio to a proper fraction, a decimal fraction, and a percent

A *ratio* is another way of indicating the relationship between the two numbers. In other words, it is another way to express a fraction. A ratio indicates *division*.

EXAMPLE: ¾ written as a ratio is 3:4
In reading a ratio the colon is read as "is to." The example would then be read as "three is to four."

EXAMPLE: 7 written as a ratio is 7:1
To express any whole number as a ratio, the number following the colon is *always* 1. The example would be read as "seven is to one."

Changing a proper fraction to a ratio reduced to lowest terms

1. Reduce the fraction to lowest terms.
2. Write the numerator of the fraction as the first number of the ratio.
3. Place a colon after the first number.
4. Write the denominator of the fraction as the second number of the ratio.

EXAMPLE: ⁴⁄₁₂
⁴⁄₁₂ reduced to lowest terms equals ⅓
⅓ written as a ratio would be 1:3

EXAMPLE: ¹⁄₁₀₀₀/¹⁄₁₀

$$\frac{1}{1000} \div \frac{1}{10} =$$

$$\frac{1}{\underset{100}{\cancel{1000}}} \times \frac{\overset{1}{\cancel{10}}}{1} = \frac{1}{100}$$

¹⁄₁₀₀₀/¹⁄₁₀ reduced to lowest terms equals ¹⁄₁₀₀
¹⁄₁₀₀ written as a ratio would be 1:100

Changing a decimal fraction to a ratio reduced to lowest terms

1. Express the decimal fraction as a proper fraction reduced to lowest terms.
2. Write the numerator of the fraction as the first number of the ratio.
3. Place a colon after the first number.
4. Write the denominator of the fraction as the second number of the ratio.

EXAMPLE: 0.85

$$\frac{85}{100} = \frac{17}{20} \text{ (reduced to lowest terms)}$$

$\frac{17}{20}$ written as a ratio would be $17:20$

EXAMPLE: 0.125

$$\frac{125}{1000} = \frac{1}{8} \text{ (reduced to lowest terms)}$$

$\frac{1}{8}$ written as a ratio would be $1:8$

Changing a percent to a ratio reduced to lowest terms

1. Express the percent as a proper fraction reduced to lowest terms.
2. Write the numerator of the fraction as the first number of the ratio.
3. Place a colon after the first number.
4. Write the denominator of the fraction as the second number of the ratio.

EXAMPLE: 30%

$$\frac{30}{100} = \frac{3}{10} \text{ (reduced to lowest terms)}$$

$\frac{3}{10}$ written as a ratio would be $3:10$

EXAMPLE: ½%

$$\frac{\frac{1}{2}}{100} =$$

$$\frac{1}{2} \div \frac{100}{1} =$$

$$\frac{1}{2} \times \frac{1}{100} = \frac{1}{200}$$

$\frac{1}{200}$ written as a ratio would be $1:200$

EXAMPLE: 3⁹/₁₀%

$$\frac{3\frac{9}{10}}{100} =$$

$$\frac{39}{10} \div \frac{100}{1} =$$

$$\frac{39}{10} \times \frac{1}{100} = \frac{39}{1000}$$

$\frac{39}{1000}$ written as a ratio would be 39:1000

Changing a ratio to a proper fraction reduced to lowest terms

1. Write the first number of the ratio as a numerator.
2. Write the second number of the ratio as the denominator.
3. Reduce the fraction to lowest terms.

EXAMPLE: 9:15   EXAMPLE: 11:22

$$\frac{9}{15} = \frac{3}{5}$$ $$\frac{11}{22} = \frac{1}{2}$$

(reduced to lowest terms)   (reduced to lowest terms)

Changing a ratio to a decimal fraction

1. Divide the first number of the ratio by the second number of the ratio, using long division.

EXAMPLE: 4:5 written as a decimal is 0.8

```
    0.8
5)4.0
  4 0
```

EXAMPLE: 3½:2¼

3.5:2.25

```
            1.555
2.25∧)3.50∧000
      2 25
      1 25 0
      1 12 5
        12 50
        11 25
         1 250
         1 125
```

3½:2¼ written as a decimal is 1.555

Changing a ratio to a percent

1. Express the ratio as a proper fraction or a decimal fraction, whichever you prefer to work with.

89

2. Multiply by 100.
3. Add the percent sign (%).

EXAMPLE: 3:5   EXAMPLE: 60:180

Changing to a proper fraction: Changing to a proper fraction:

$$\frac{3}{5} \times \frac{\overset{20}{\cancel{100}}}{1} = \frac{60}{1}$$

$$\frac{60}{180} = \frac{1}{3}$$

60 + % = 60%.

$$\frac{1}{3} \times \frac{100}{1} = \frac{100}{3} = 33\frac{1}{3}$$

Changing to a decimal fraction:

$33\frac{1}{3} + \% = 33\frac{1}{3}\%$

$$5\overline{)\begin{array}{l}0.6 \\ 3.0\end{array}}$$
$$\underline{3\ 0}$$

Changing to a decimal fraction:

$$180\overline{)\begin{array}{l}0.333 \\ 60.000\end{array}}$$
$$\underline{54\ 0}$$
$$6\ 00$$
$$\underline{5\ 40}$$
$$600$$
$$\underline{540}$$
$$600$$
$$\underline{540}$$
$$60$$

$0.6 \times 100 = 60$

$60 + \% = 60\%$

$0.333 \times 100 = 33.3$

$33.3 + \% = 33.3\%$

Study the introductory material. The processes for the calculation of the problems are listed in steps. Memorize the steps for each calculation before beginning the work sheet. Complete the following work sheet that provides for extensive practice in the manipulation of ratios. Check your answers. If you have difficulties, go back and review the steps for that type of calculation. When you feel ready to evaluate your learning, take the first posttest. Check your answers. An acceptable score as indicated on the posttest signifies that you are ready for the next chapter. An unacceptable score signifies a need for further study before taking the second posttest.

CHAPTER 4
RATIOS

WORK SHEET

Change the following fractions to ratios reduced to lowest terms.

1. $\frac{3}{4}$

2. $\frac{1}{3}$

3. $\frac{9}{12}$

4. $\frac{4}{6}$

5. $\frac{3}{10}$

6. $\frac{11}{22}$

7. $\frac{6}{9}$

8. $\frac{56}{100}$

9. $\frac{6}{24}$

10. $\frac{20}{50}$

11. $\frac{310}{1000}$

12. $\frac{17}{34}$

13. $\frac{10}{16}$

14. $\frac{3}{8}/\frac{1}{4}$

15. $2\frac{1}{2}/1\frac{3}{4}$

16. $5/6 / 3\frac{1}{3}$

17. $4\frac{3}{16} / \frac{7}{8}$

18. $1\frac{3}{5} / 2\frac{7}{10}$

19. $\frac{1}{10} / \frac{1}{100}$

20. $1\frac{4}{30} / 2$

21. $3/67$

22. $1\frac{24}{38} / 2\frac{4}{10}$

23. $3\frac{1}{3} / 3\frac{1}{3}$

24. $5/8 / 2\frac{4}{5}$

Change the following decimal fractions to ratios reduced to lowest terms.

1. 0.896

2. 0.96

3. 0.6738

4. 0.06

5. 0.756

6. 0.6

7. 0.4032

8. 0.821

9. 0.74

10. 0.166

11. 0.4376

12. 0.26

13. 0.492

14. 0.33

15. 0.820

16. 0.95

17. 0.2

18. 0.235

19. 0.67

20. 0.5355

21. 0.846

22. 0.172

23. 0.9

24. 0.4752

Change the following percents to ratios reduced to lowest terms.

1. 10%

2. 2½%

3. 33⅓%

4. ⅜%

5. 25%

6. 2⁷⁄₁₀%

7. 44%

8. 15.7%

9. 4⅘%

10. 55.62%

11. 7¾%

12. 35%

13. 2.5%

14. 0.44%

15. 0.05%

16. 7.8%

17. 1%

18. 6¾%

19. 9⅝%

20. 0.14%

21. ⅗%

22. 12⅑%

23. 3³⁄₇%

24. 8.2%

Change the following ratios to fractions reduced to lowest terms.

1. 1:2

2. 3:4

3. 4:64

4. 8:10

5. 4:800

6. 3:150

7. 9:300

8. ⅜:¼

9. 9:27

10. 4/7:⅖

11. 8/12:⅔

12. 2½:7½

13. ⅘:¼

14. 1/10::4/20

15. 12:60

16. $^4/_{75} : {}^3/_{10}$ **17.** $1^5/_{21} : 2^3/_7$ **18.** $0.25 : 0.75$

19. $0.68 : 0.44$ **20.** $1.85 : 3.35$ **21.** $0.4 : 0.126$

22. $0.7 : 42.9$ **23.** $1.64 : 2.54$ **24.** $1.21 : 8.21$

Change the following ratios to decimal numbers.

1. $7 : 14$ **2.** $5 : 20$ **3.** $3 : 8$

4. $20 : 32$ **5.** $11 : 33$ **6.** $^5/_8 : {}^1/_{10}$

7. $^1/_{1000} : {}^1/_{500}$ **8.** $^3/_4 : {}^1/_2$ **9.** $^1/_{75} : {}^3/_{15}$

10. ³⁄₁₀₀₀ : ³⁄₁₀₀ **11.** 2 : 5 **12.** 0.105 : 0.232

13. 6½ : 12¾ **14.** ½ : ⁵⁄₉ **15.** ⅙ : ⅝

16. 2⁵⁄₁₆ : 4⁵⁄₁₂ **17.** 7 : 259 **18.** 0.42 : 0.88

19. 0.91 : 2.34 **20.** 62.4 : 0.01 **21.** 3.5 : 1.2

22. 4.8 : 0.4 **23.** 7 : 9 **24.** 1²⁄₅ : ¹²⁄₃₀

Change the following ratios to percents.

1. 2 : 4 **2.** 7 : 231 **3.** 25 : 250

4. 30:150   **5.** ⁶/₇:⅔   **6.** ¾:1¹/₂₀

7. 1¼:3⅜   **8.** 0.35:0.2   **9.** 1:1000

10. 0.15:0.6   **11.** 0.85:1.50   **12.** 5½:2⅔

13. ⁵/₁₆:⅗   **14.** ³/₂₅:⁴/₇₅   **15.** 1:500

16. 1⁸/₁₂:2³/₆   **17.** 19:20   **18.** ⁴/₁₁:1½

19. 2.5 : 4.5   **20.** 12 : 38   **21.** 32 : 160

22. 4 : ³⁄₁₆   **23.** 5.2 : 2.3   **24.** 13 : 23

Answers on pp. 352-353.

Name _____

Date _____

ACCEPTABLE SCORE __27__

YOUR SCORE _____

POSTTEST 1

DIRECTIONS: Convert to equivalents.

	Ratio	Fraction	Decimal	Percent
1	42.48			
2			0.004	
3		$^{13}/_{20}$		
4				$2\frac{1}{4}\%$
5			0.35	
6		$^{6}/_{25}$		
7	$^{3}/_{8} : ^{5}/_{9}$			
8				0.3%
9			0.205	
10		$^{4}/_{11}$		

Answers on p. 353.

Name _____

Date _____

POSTTEST 2

DIRECTIONS: Convert to equivalents.

	Ratio	**Fraction**	**Decimal**	**Percent**
1	7:10			
2		5/16		
3			0.075	
4				6%
5				3/8%
6		1/150		
7			0.007	
8	6:21			
9			0.322	
10				18.2%

Answers on p. 353.

Name _____

Date _____

ACCEPTABLE SCORE __**18**__

YOUR SCORE _____

PRETEST

DIRECTIONS: Find the value of x. Show your work.

1. $25:75::x:300$

2. $450:15::225:x$

3. $x:\frac{1}{4}\%::8:12$

4. $12:3::x:0.8$

5. $0.6:2.4::32:x$

6. $150:x::75:2$

7. $\frac{1}{8}:\frac{2}{3}::75:x$

8. $\frac{1}{200}:8::x:800$

9. $x:\frac{1}{2}::\frac{3}{4}:\frac{7}{8}$

10. $16:x::24:12$

11. $\frac{2}{3}:\frac{1}{5}::x:24$

12. $x:9::\frac{2}{3}:36$

13. $\frac{1}{7}:x::\frac{1}{2}:49$

14. $0.8:4::9.6:x$

15. $\frac{4}{5}:x::\frac{2}{3}:\frac{1}{4}$

16. $40:80::x:160$ **17.** $2.5:x::4:16$ **18.** $8:72::14:x$

19. $x:\frac{1}{15}::50:500$ **20.** $5:100::x:325$

Answers on p. 353.

CHAPTER 5
PROPORTIONS

Learning objectives _____

On completion of the materials provided in this chapter, you will be able to perform computations accurately by mastering the following mathematical concepts:

1. Solving simple proportion problems
2. Solving proportion problems involving fractions, decimals, and percents

A proportion consists of two ratios of equal value. The ratios are connected by a double colon ($::$) which symbolizes the word "as."

$$2:3::4:6$$

Read the above proportion: "Two is to three as four is to six."

The first and fourth terms of the proportion are the extremes. The second and third terms are the means.

$$2:3::4:6$$

2 and 6 are the extremes.
3 and 4 are the means.

In a proportion, the product of the means equals the product of the extremes because the ratios are of equal value. This principle may be used to verify your answer in a proportion problem.

$$3 \times 4 = 12, \text{ means}$$
$$2 \times 6 = 12, \text{ extremes}$$

If three terms in the proportions are known and one term is unknown, an x is inserted in the space for the unknown term.

$$2:3::4:x$$

SOLVING A SIMPLE PROPORTION PROBLEM

1. Multiply the means.
2. Multiply the extremes.
3. Place the product including the x on the *left* and the product of the known terms on the *right*.
4. Divide the product of the known terms by the number next to x. The quotient will be the value of x.

Proportion problem involving whole numbers

EXAMPLE:

$$2:3::4:x$$

$$2x = 3 \times 4$$

$$2x = 12$$

$$x = 12 \div 2$$

$$x = 6$$

Proportion problem involving fractions

EXAMPLE:

$$\frac{1}{150}:\frac{1}{100}::x:60$$

$$\frac{1}{100x} = \frac{1}{150} \times 60$$

$$\frac{1}{100x} = \frac{2}{5}$$

$$x = \frac{2}{5} \div \frac{1}{100}$$

$$x = \frac{2}{\cancel{5}} \times \frac{\cancel{100}^{20}}{1}$$
$$_{1}$$

$$x = 40$$

Proportion problem involving decimals

EXAMPLE:

$$0.4:0.8::0.25:x$$

$$0.4x = 0.8 \times 0.25$$

$$0.4x = 0.2$$

$$x = 0.2 \div 0.4$$

$$x = 0.5$$

Proportion problem involving fractions and percents

EXAMPLE: $x : \frac{1}{4}\% : : 9\frac{3}{5} : \frac{1}{200}$

Convert $\frac{1}{4}\%$ to a proper fraction and $9\frac{3}{5}$ to an improper fraction. Then, rewrite the proportion using these fractions.

$$x : \frac{1}{400} : : \frac{48}{5} : \frac{1}{200}$$

$$\frac{1}{200x} = \frac{1}{400} \times \frac{48}{5}$$

$$\frac{1}{200x} = \frac{3}{125}$$

$$x = \frac{3}{125} \div \frac{1}{200}$$

$$x = \frac{3}{\cancel{125}_{5}} \times \frac{\cancel{200}^{8}}{1}$$

$$x = \frac{24}{5}$$

$$x = 4\frac{4}{5}$$

Proportion problem involving decimals and percents

EXAMPLE: $0.3\% : 1.8 : : x : 14.4$

Convert 0.3% to a decimal

$$0.003 : 1.8 = x : 14.4$$

$$1.8x = 0.003 \times 14.4$$

$$1.8x = 0.0432$$

$$x = 0.0432 \div 1.8$$

$$x = 0.024$$

Proportion problem involving numerous zeros

EXAMPLE: $250{,}000 : x : : 500{,}000 : 4$

$$500{,}000x = 250{,}000 \times 4$$

$$500{,}000x = 1{,}000{,}000$$

$$x = 1{,}000{,}000 \div 500{,}000$$

$$\text{or } x = \frac{1{,}000{,}000}{500{,}000}$$

$$x = 2$$

Most problems concerning drug dosage can be solved by a proportion problem, whether it involves fractions, decimals, or percents. If a proportion problem contains any combination of fractions, decimals, or percents, all forms within the problems must be converted to either fractions or decimals.

Study the introductory material. The process for the calculation of proportion problems is listed in steps. Memorize the steps before beginning the work sheet. Complete the following work sheet, which provides for extensive practice in the manipulation of proportions. Check your answers. If you have difficulties, go back and review the necessary steps. When you feel ready to evaluate your learning, take the first posttest. Check your answers. An acceptable score as indicated on the posttest signifies that you are ready for the next chapter. An unacceptable score signifies a need for further study before taking the second posttest.

WORK SHEET

Find the value of x. Show your work.

1. $20:400::x:1680$

2. $100:x::64:384$

3. $0.9:2.4::x:75$

4. $\frac{5}{6}:x::\frac{5}{9}:\frac{4}{5}$

5. $3:90::1\frac{3}{4}:x$

6. $2:3::18:x$

7. $\frac{1}{300}:4::6:x$

8. $75:x::100:2$

9. $\frac{1}{6}:1::\frac{1}{8}:x$

10. $200,000:x::1,000,000:5$

11. $x:\frac{3}{4}\%::3\frac{1}{5}:\frac{1}{200}$

12. $84:x::30:90$

13. $24:x::6:60$

14. $\frac{1}{150}:1::\frac{1}{100}:x$

15. $3:150::40:x$

16. $\frac{1}{8}:x::7:56$ **17.** $\frac{1}{200}:40::\frac{1}{100}:x$ **18.** $x:5::3:15$

19. $9:x::3:800$ **20.** $15:60::x:20$ **21.** $12\frac{1}{2}:x::50:2400$

22. $\frac{1}{2}\%:\frac{1}{100}::x:80$ **23.** $x:6.4::0.03:6$ **24.** $15:16::120:x$

25. $0.25:1::0.05:x$ **26.** $7:14::x:16$ **27.** $x:8::6:96$

28. $\frac{1}{120}:2::4:x$ **29.** $x:\frac{1}{1000}::5:\frac{1}{5000}$ **30.** $6:15::8:x$

31. $x:3::9:54$ **32.** $1.4:0.4::4.2:x$ **33.** $x:0.65::9:5$

34. $12\frac{1}{2}\%:5::x:120$

35. $\frac{1}{300}:6::\frac{1}{120}:x$

36. $x:45::4:6$

37. $25:75::16:x$

38. $30:90::5:x$

39. $0.3:x::7:21$

40. $20:25::x:5$

41. $x:12::9:6$

42. $4:x::12:48$

43. $x:60::900:40$

44. $x:12::2:4$

45. $6:20::x:120$

46. $\frac{4}{5}:x::\frac{1}{3}:\frac{5}{9}$

47. $25:50::4:x$

48. $0.6:x::7:42$

49. $15:x::20:600$

50. $0.6:x::0.4:12$

51. $9\%:x::11:73$

52. $500,000:1::300,000:x$

53. $\frac{1}{6}:\frac{9}{10}::\frac{1}{2}:x$

54. $2.5:x::0.5:400$

55. $2.8:12::40:x$

56. $8:\frac{8}{100}::x:5$

57. $\frac{1}{8}\%:\frac{1}{200}::x:40$

58. $x:25::18:36$

59. $0.15:0.25::x:400$

60. $\frac{1}{20}:\frac{1}{15}::x:25$

61. $800,000:5::960,000:x$

62. $0.50:0.40::x:400$

63. $83.25:60::x:45$

64. $27:x::9:60$

65. $\frac{1}{20}:\frac{1}{5}::x:50$

66. $\frac{1}{150}:\frac{1}{200}::x:60$

67. $\frac{1}{2}\% : 4 :: x : 25$ **68.** $0.6 : 1.2 :: x : 200$ **69.** $500 : 2.5 :: x : 8.1$

70. $x : 80 :: 14 : 56$

Answers on pp. 353-354.

POSTTEST 1

DIRECTIONS: **Find the value of x. Show your work.**

1. $x:2.5::4:5$

2. $7/8:x::4/5:2/3$

3. $30:90::2:x$

4. $x:3.5::25:14$

5. $2/7:1/2::x:56$

6. $1/4:x::160:320$

7. $x:7::5:14$

8. $3:x::18:12$

9. $1/5:90::x:250$

10. $1.8:4.8::x:96$

11. $x:8::10:20$

12. $2/3:x::4.5:27$

13. $1/150:x::1/200:6$

14. $2/3\%:1/5::50:x$

15. $14:x::6:18$

16. $x : \frac{2}{3} :: 12 : 18$

17. $50 : 250 :: \frac{4}{5} : x$

18. $50 : 3 :: x : 6$

19. $\frac{1}{2} : x :: 40 : 80$

20. $0.8 : 10 :: x : 40$

Answers on p. 354.

POSTTEST 2

DIRECTIONS: Find the value of x. Show your work.

1. $x:300::9:12$

2. $4:32\%::16:x$

3. $18:x::6:40$

4. $1.8:2.5::x:9.5$

5. $x:30::\frac{1}{3}:\frac{3}{4}$

6. $\frac{7}{8}:x::\frac{5}{8}:40$

7. $400:500::\frac{4}{5}:x$

8. $x:7.6::3:6$

9. $\frac{1}{4}:x::\frac{2}{3}:\frac{2}{5}$

10. $\frac{1}{150}:\frac{1}{100}::x:60$

11. $0.6:x::15:90$

12. $3.5:12::x:360$

13. $\frac{2}{9}:\frac{4}{5}::\frac{3}{4}:x$

14. $\frac{1}{8}:x::\frac{1}{7}:\frac{5}{9}$

15. $x:2.5::16:4$

16. $0.6:3::72:x$ **17.** $20:x::6:4.5$ **18.** $x:\frac{1}{4}::96:\frac{1}{3}$

19. $300:5000::x:18$ **20.** $\frac{1}{3}:x::\frac{1}{5}:90$

Answers on p. 354.

PART II

Units and measures for the calculation of drug dosages

PRETEST

DIRECTIONS: Change to equivalents within the apothecaries' system. Solve by using proportions. Show your work.

1. 20 gr = _____ ʒ

2. 360 gr = _____ ʒ = _____ ℥

3. 72 ʒ = _____ ℥ = _____ gr

4. 10 ℥ = _____ gr = _____ ʒ

5. 120 ℳ = _____ fl ʒ = _____ fl ℥

6. 300 ℳ = _____ fl ʒ = _____ fl ℥

7. 12½ fl ʒ = _____ fl ℥ = _____ ℳ

8. 160 fl ʒ = _____ fl ℥ = _____ pt = _____ qt

9. 12 fl ℥ = _____ fl ʒ = _____ pt

10. 64 fl ℥ = _____ fl ʒ = _____ pt = _____ qt

11. 5 pt = _____ fl ℥ = _____ fl ʒ = _____ qt

12. 1¼ pt = _____ ♏ = _____ fl ℥ = _____ fl ʒ

13. 7 qt = _____ gal = _____ fl ʒ

14. 2½ qt = _____ fl ℥ = _____ fl ʒ = _____ pt

15. 1¼ gal = _____ qt = _____ pt = _____ fl ʒ

DIRECTIONS: Change the following household measurements into approximate equivalents within the apothecaries' system. Solve the problem by the use of a proportion. Show your work.

16. 3 glasses = _____ fl ℥

17. 1½ Tbsp. = _____ fl ʒ

18. 10 gtt = _____ ♍

19. 1¾ tsp = _____ fl ʒ

20. 2½ cups = _____ fl ℥

Answers on p. 354.

CHAPTER 6

APOTHECARIES' AND HOUSEHOLD MEASUREMENTS

Learning objectives

On completion of the materials provided in this chapter, you will be able to perform computations accurately by mastering the following mathematical concepts:

1. Addition and subtraction of roman numerals
2. Conversion of roman numerals to arabic numerals
3. Conversion of arabic numerals to roman numerals
4. Recall of the apothecaries' measures of weights and liquids
5. Computation of equivalents within the apothecaries' system by the use of a proportion
6. Recall of approximate equivalents between apothecaries' and household measures
7. Computation of equivalents between the apothecaries' and household measurement systems by the use of a proportion

The apothecaries' system of measure is very old. When writing orders in the apothecaries' system, physicians usually utilize roman numerals. All parts of a whole are expressed as a fraction except the fraction one-half, which is commonly represented as $\overline{ss}$.

The following is a list of the more frequently used roman numerals and their arabic equivalents. Memorize the list.

Roman numeral	Arabic numeral
i	1
v	5
x	10
l	50
c	100

Only addition and subtraction may be performed in the roman numeral system.

Addition of roman numerals

1. Addition is performed when a smaller numeral follows a larger numeral.

EXAMPLES: xi = 11   xv = 15   li = 51

2. Addition is performed when a numeral is repeated. However, a numeral is *never* repeated more than three times.

EXAMPLE: viii = 8   xii = 12   ccxi = 211

Subtraction of roman numerals

1. Subtraction is performed when a smaller numeral is placed before a larger numeral.

   EXAMPLES: ix = 9   iv = 4   ic = 99

2. Subtraction is performed when a smaller numeral is placed between two larger numerals. The smaller numeral is subtracted from the larger numeral following the smaller numeral.

   EXAMPLES: xiv = 14   xxiv = 24   cxc = 190

Apothecaries' measurements

The nurse is already familiar with many of the units of measure in the apothecaries' system because they are used every day; a nurse most frequently uses the following list of apothecaries' system units of measure. Memorize all entries in the list.

Apothecaries' measure of weight

60 grains (gr) = 1 dram (ʒ)

8 drams (ʒ) = 1 ounce (℥)

Apothcaries' measure of liquid

60 minims (♏) = 1 fluidram (fl ʒ)

8 fluidrams (fl ʒ) = 1 fluidounce (fl ℥)

16 fluidounces (fl ℥) = 1 pint (pt)

32 fluidounces (fl ℥) = 2 pints (pt) or 1 quart (qt)

4 quarts (qt) = 1 gallon (gal)

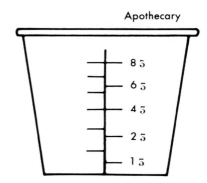

Apothecary

Sometimes, to compute drug dosages, it is necessary for the nurse to convert an apothecaries' measure to an equivalent measure within the same system. This may easily be done by the use of a proportion.

EXAMPLE: 3 fl ℥ equals how many fl ʒ?

a. On the left side of the proportion, place what you know to be an equivalent between fluidrams and fluidounces. From the preceding chart you know that there are 8 fl ʒ in 1 fl ℥. Therefore the left side of the proportion would be

8 fl ʒ:1 fl ℥::

b. What will be on the right side of the proportion is determined by the problem and by the abbreviations used on the left side of the proportion. Only *two* different abbreviations may be used in a single proportion. The abbreviations must also be in the same position on the right as they are on the left.

8 fl ʒ:1 fl ℥:: _____ fl ʒ: _____ fl ℥

From the problem we know we have 3 fl ℥.

$$8 \text{ fl } ℥:1 \text{ fl } ʒ::\underline{\hspace{2cm}} \text{ fl } ʒ:3 \text{ fl } ℥$$

Since we need to find the number of fluidrams 3 fl ℥ equals, we use the symbol x to represent the unknown. Therefore the full proportion would be written as follows:

$$8 \text{ fl } ℥:1 \text{ fl } ʒ::x \text{ fl } ʒ:3 \text{ fl } ℥$$

c. Rewrite the proportion without using the abbreviations.

$$8:1::x:3$$

d. Solve for x.

$$1x = 8 \times 3$$
$$x = 24$$

e. Label your answer, as determined by the abbreviation placed next to x in the original proportion.

$$3 \text{ fl } ℥ = 24 \text{ fl } ʒ$$

EXAMPLE: 12 fl ℥ equals how many pints?

a. 16 fl ℥:1 pt::
b. 16 fl ℥:1 pt:: \underline{\hspace{2cm}} fl ℥: \underline{\hspace{2cm}} pt
   16 fl ℥:1 pt ::12 fl ℥:x pt
c. 16:1::12:x
d. 16x = 12
$$x = \frac{12}{16} = \frac{3}{4}$$
e. 12 fl ℥ equals ¾ pt

EXAMPLE: 1 ½ fl ʒ = \underline{\hspace{2cm}} ♏

a. 60 ♏:1 fl ʒ ::
b. 60 ♏:1 fl ʒ :: \underline{\hspace{2cm}} ♏: \underline{\hspace{2cm}} fl ʒ
   60 ♏:1 fl ʒ :: x♏: 1 ½ fl ʒ
c. 60:1::x:1 ½
d. 1x = 60 × 1 ½
$$x = \frac{\overset{30}{\cancel{60}}}{1} \times \frac{3}{\underset{1}{\cancel{2}}}$$
$$x = 90$$
e. 1 ½ fl ʒ = 90 ♏

Household measurements

Household measures are not accurate enough to be used by the nurse in the calculation of drug dosages in the hospital. It is sometimes necessary to compute their approximate equivalents with the apothecaries' system of measure, especially when sending medicines home from the hospital.

Memorize the following list of approximate equivalents.

Apothecaries' measures Household measures

1 minim ($\mathfrak{m}$) = 1 drop (gtt)
1 fluidram (fl ℨ) = 1 teaspoon (tsp)
4 fluidrams (fl ℨ) = 1 tablespoon (Tbsp)
6 fluidounces (fl ℥) = 1 cup (c)
8 fluidounces (fl℥) = 1 glass

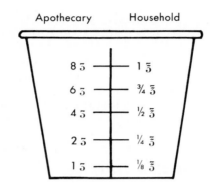

Conversion of measures between the apothecaries' and household systems of measure may also be made by the use of a proportion, as has been illustrated.

EXAMPLE: 1 ½ c equals how many fl ℥?

a. **6 fl ℥:1 c::**
b. **6 fl ℥: 1 c:: _____ fl ℥ _____ c**
   6 fl ℥:1 c::x fl ℥: 1 ½ c
c. **6:1::x:1 ½**
d.
$$x = \frac{\overset{3}{\cancel{6}}}{1} \times \frac{3}{\underset{1}{\cancel{2}}}$$

$$x = \frac{18}{2} = 9$$

e. **1 ½ c = 9 fl ℥**

EXAMPLE: 2 tsp = _____ fl ℥

a. **1 fl ℥:1 tsp ::**
b. **1 fl ℥:1 tsp :: _____ fl ℥: _____ tsp**
   1 fl ℥:1 tsp::x fl ℥:2 tsp
c. **1:1::x:2**
d. **1x = 2**
   x = 2
e. **2 tsp = 2 fl ℥**

Memorize the tables for the apothecaries' and household measurements. Study the material on forming proportions for the calculation of problems relating to the apothecaries' and household systems of measure. Complete the following work sheet, which provides for extensive practice in the manipulation of measurements within the apothecaries' and household systems. Check your answers. If you have difficulties, go back and review the necessary material. When you feel ready to evaluate your learning, take the first posttest. Check your answers. An acceptable score as indicated on the posttest signifies that you are ready for the next chapter. An unacceptable score signifies a need for further study before taking the second posttest.

APOTHECARIES' AND
HOUSEHOLD MEASUREMENTS

WORK SHEET

Express the following arabic numerals in roman numerals.

1. 22   **2.** 9   **3.** 43   **4.** 3

5. 160   **6.** 18   **7.** 30   **8.** 210

9. 14   **10.** 67   **11.** 15   **12.** 21

13. 12   **14.** 27   **15.** 49

Express the following roman numerals in arabic numerals.

1. xxix   **2.** lxiv   **3.** vii   **4.** lvii

5. civ   **6.** xxxiv   **7.** vi   **8.** xiii

9. xix   **10.** xxxviii   **11.** xl   **12.** iv

13. xxv   **14.** xxxix   **15.** ccxl

Change to equivalents within the apothecaries' system. Solve, using proportions. Show your work.

1. 30 gr = _____ ℥

2. 180 gr = _____ ℥ = _____ ℥

3. 740 gr = _____ ℥ = _____ ℥

4. ⅓ ℥ = _____ gr

5. 16 ℥ = _____ ℥ = _____ gr

6. 520 ℥ = _____ ℥ = _____ gr

7. 60 ℨ = _____ ℥ = _____ gr   **8.** 90 ♏ = _____ fl ℨ = _____ fl ℥

9. 240 ♏ = _____ fl ℨ = _____ fl ℥   **10.** 510 ♏ = _____ fl ℨ = _____ fl ℥ = _____ pt

11. 20 ♏ = _____ fl ℨ   **12.** 720 ♏ = _____ fl ℥

13. 10 fl ℨ = _____ fl ℥ = _____ ♏   **14.** 20 fl ℨ = _____ fl ℥ = _____ pt = _____ ♏

15. 6 ½ fl ℨ = _____ fl ℥ = _____ ♏   **16.** 120 fl ℨ = _____ fl ℥ = _____ pt = _____ qt

17. 64 fl ℨ = _____ fl ℥ = _____ pt = _____ qt   **18.** 3 pt = _____ ♏ = _____ fl ℨ = _____ fl ℥

19. 4 pt = _____ fl ℨ = _____ fl ℥ = _____ qt

20. 2 ½ pt = _____ fl ℥ = _____ fl ℨ = _____ ᴍ

21. 8 pt = _____ qt = _____ gal

22. ½ pt = _____ ᴍ = _____ fl ℥ = _____ fl ℨ

23. 3 qt = _____ gal = _____ fl ℥ = _____ pt

24. 10 qt = _____ pt = _____ fl ℨ = _____ gal

25. 1 ½ gal = _____ qt = _____ pt = _____ fl ℨ

Change the following household measurements into appropriate equivalents within the apothecaries' system. Solve the problems by the use of proportions. Show your work.

26. 2 tsp = _____ fl ℨ

27. 4 tsp = _____ fl ℨ

28. 3 Tbsp = _____ fl ʒ = _____ fl ʒ

29. 2 ½ Tbsp = _____ fl ʒ = _____ fl ʒ

30. 1 ¾ cup = _____ fl ʒ = _____ fl ʒ

31. 2 glasses = _____ fl ʒ

32. 10 gtt = _____ ♏

33. ½ cup = _____ fl ʒ = _____ fl ʒ

34. 3 ¼ glasses = _____ fl ʒ = _____ fl ʒ

Answers on pp. 354-355.

134

Name _____

Date _____

ACCEPTABLE SCORE ____36____

YOUR SCORE _____

POSTTEST 1

DIRECTIONS: **Change to equivalents within the apothecaries' system. Solve by using proportions. Show your work.**

1. 45 gr = _____ ℨ

2. 240 gr = _____ ℨ = _____ ℥

3. 360 ℨ = _____ ℥ = _____ gr

4. 68 ℨ = _____ fl ℥ = _____ gr

5. 4 ℥ = _____ gr = _____ ℨ

6. 100 ♏ = _____ ℨ = _____ fl ℥

7. 320 ♏ = _____ fl ℨ = _____ fl ℥

8. 40 fl ℨ = _____ fl ℥ = _____ ♏ = _____ pt

9. 180 fl ℥ _____ fl ʒ = _____ pt = _____ qt

10. 10 fl ℥ = _____ fl ʒ = _____ pt

11. 48 fl ℥ = _____ fl ʒ = _____ pt = _____ qt

12. 3 ½ pt = _____ fl ℥ = _____ fl ʒ

13. ¾ pt = _____ fl ℥ = _____ fl ℥

14. 5 qt = _____ gal = _____ pt = _____ fl ℥ = _____ fl ℥

15. 1 ¾ gal = _____ qt = _____ pt = _____ fl ℥

DIRECTIONS: Change the following household measurements into approximate equivalents within the apothecaries' system. Solve the problem by the use of a proportion. Show your work.

16. 1 ½ glasses = _____ fl ℥

17. ¾ cup = _____ fl ℥

18. 3 Tbsp = _____ fl ℥

19. 2 ½ tsp = _____ fl ℥

20. 20 gtt = _____ ♏

Answers on p. 355.

Name _____

Date _____

ACCEPTABLE SCORE ___36___

YOUR SCORE _____

POSTTEST 2

DIRECTIONS: Change to equivalents within the apothecaries' system. Solve by using proportions. Show your work.

1. 15 gr = _____ ʒ

2. 300 gr = _____ ʒ = _____ ℥

3. 480 ʒ = _____ ℥ = _____ gr

4. 6 ℥ = _____ gr = _____ ʒ

5. 110 ♏ = _____ fl ʒ = _____ fl ℥

6. 330 ♏ = _____ fl ʒ = _____ fl ℥

7. 30 fl ʒ = _____ fl ℥ = _____ ♏ = _____ pt

8. 210 fl ʒ = _____ fl ℥ = _____ pt = _____ qt

9. 14 fl ℥ = _____ fl ℈ = _____ pt

10. 72 fl ℥ = _____ fl ℈ = _____ pt = _____ qt

11. 4 ½ pt = _____ fl ℥ = _____ ℈

12. ¼ pt = _____ ♏ = _____ fl ℈ = _____ fl ℥

13. 6 qt = _____ gal = _____ fl ℥

14. 3 ¼ qt = _____ fl ℈ = _____ fl ℥ = _____ pt

15. 2 ½ gal = _____ qt = _____ pt = _____ fl ℥

DIRECTIONS: Change the following household measurements into approximate equivalents within the apothecaries' system. Solve the problem by the use of a proportion. Show your work.

16. 5 Tbsp = _____ fl ℈

17. 2 ¼ cup = _____ fl ℥

18. ½ glass = _____ fl ℥

19. 3 tsp = _____ fl ℥

20. 5 gtt = _____ ♏

Answers on p. 355.

Name _____

Date _____

ACCEPTABLE SCORE ___**27**___

YOUR SCORE _____

PRETEST

DIRECTIONS: Change to equivalent metric measurements. Solve each problem by the use of a proportion. Show your work.

1. 800,000 mcg = _____ Gm

2. 3 mg = _____ mcg

3. 255 mg = _____ Gm

4. 3 Tbsp = _____ ml

5. 3000 mcg = _____ mg

6. 0.68 Gm = _____ mg

7. 326 ml = _____ L

8. 33 kg = _____ lb

9. 2.1 kl = _____ L

10. 3000 Gm = _____ kg

11. 0.1 L = _____ ml

12. 2½ tsp = _____ ml

13. 5 ml = _____ cc

14. 0.8 kg = _____ Gm

15. 250 L = _____ kl

16. 1¼ glass = _____ ml

17. 22 lb = _____ Gm

18. 0.63 L = _____ ml

19. 733 Gm = _____ kg

20. 1.25 Gm = _____ mcg

21. 60 gtt = _____ ml

22. 0.25 mg = _____ mcg

23. 0.6 kl = _____ L

24. 45 lb = _____ kg

25. 10,000 mcg = _____ Gm

26. 1.2 kg = _____ Gm

27. 1⅔ c = _____ ml

28. 0.71 Gm = _____ mg

29. 480 ml = _____ L

30. 650 Gm = _____ lb

Answers on p. 355.

METRIC AND HOUSEHOLD MEASUREMENTS

Learning objectives

On completion of the materials provided in this chapter, you will perform computations accurately by mastering the following mathematical concepts:

1. Recall of the metric measures of weights and liquids
2. Computation of equivalents within the metric system by the use of a proportion
3. Recall of approximate equivalents between metric and household measures
4. Computation of equivalents between the metric and household systems of measure by the use of a proportion

Metric measurements

The metric system is much newer than the apothecaries' system of measure. The metric system is fast becoming the system of choice when dealing with weights and measures in the area of drug dosages. This is a result of its accuracy and simplicity, since it is based on the decimal system. The use of decimals tends to eliminate the errors made when working with fractions. Certain prefixes identify the multiples of 10 that are being utilized.

The three most commonly used prefixes of the metric system involved with the calculation of drug dosages are the following: micro—one millionth, or 0.000001; milli—one thousandth, or 0.001; and kilo—1000 times.

A nurse most frequently uses the following list of metric measures. Memorize all the entries in the list.

Metric measure of weight

1,000,000 micrograms (mcg) = 1 gram (Gm)
1000 micrograms (mcg) = 1 milligram (mg)
1000 milligrams (mg) = 1 gram (Gm)
1000 grams (Gm) = 1 kilogram (kg)

Metric measure of liquid

1000 milliliters (ml) = 1 liter (L)
1000 liters (L) = 1 kiloliter (kl)
1 cubic centimeter (cc) = 1 milliliter (ml)

The cubic centimeter (cc) and the milliliter (ml) are used interchangeably. However, in this book, the millilter will be used exclusively.

Sometimes, to compute drug dosages, it is necessary for the nurse to convert a metric measure to an equivalent measure within the system. This may easily be done by the use of a proportion.

EXAMPLE: 300 mg equals how many Gm?

a. On the left side of the proportion place what you know to be an equivalent between milligrams and grams. From the preceding chart we know that there are 1000 mg in 1 Gm. Therefore the left side of the proportion would be

$$1000 \text{ mg}: 1 \text{ Gm}::$$

b. What will be the right side of the proportion will be determined by the problem and by the abbreviations used on the left side of the proportion. Only *two* different abbreviations may be used in a single proportion. The abbreviations must also be in the same position on the right as they are on the left.

$$1000 \text{ mg}: 1 \text{ Gm}:: \underline{\hspace{1cm}} \text{ mg}: \underline{\hspace{1cm}} \text{ Gm}$$

From the problem we know we have 300 mg

$$1000 \text{ mg}: 1 \text{ Gm}::300 \text{ mg}: \underline{\hspace{1cm}} \text{ Gm}$$

Since we need to find the number of grams 300 mg equals, we use the symbol x to represent the unknown. Therefore the full proportion would be

$$1000 \text{ mg}: 1 \text{ Gm}::300 \text{ mg}:x \text{ Gm}$$

c. Rewrite the proportion without using the abbreviations.

$$1000:1::300:x$$

d. Solve for x, writing the answer as a decimal, since the metric system is based on decimals.

$$1000x = 300$$
$$x = \frac{300}{1000}$$
$$x = 0.3$$

e. Label your answer, as determined by the abbreviation placed next to x in the original proportion.

$$300 \text{ mg} = 0.3 \text{ Gm}$$

EXAMPLE: 2.5 L equals how many milliliters?

a. 1000 ml: 1L::
b. 1000 ml:1 L:: \underline{\hspace{1cm}} ml: \underline{\hspace{1cm}} L
   1000 ml:1 L::x ml:2.5L
c. 1000:1::x:2.5
d. 1x = 2500
   x = 2500
e. 2.5 L equals 2500 ml

EXAMPLE: 180 mcg equals how many grams?

a. 1,000,000 mcg:1 Gm::
b. 1,000,000 mcg:1 Gm:: \underline{\hspace{1cm}} mcg: \underline{\hspace{1cm}} Gm
   1,000,000 mcg: 1 Gm::180 mcg:x Gm
c. 1,000,000:1::180:x

d. 1,000,000 $x = 180$

           $x = 0.00018$

e. 180 mcg equals 0.00018 Gm

Household measurements

Household measures are not accurate enough for the nurse to use in the calculation of drug dosages in the hospital. However, their metric equivalents are used in keeping a written record of a patient's "I" and "O," or intake and output.

Memorize the following list of approximate equivalents between metric and household measurements.

Metric measure		Household measure
1 milliliter (ml)	=	15 drops (gtt)
4 milliliters	=	1 teaspoon (tsp)
15 milliliters	=	1 tablespoon (Tbsp)
180 milliliters	=	1 cup (c)
240 milliliters	=	1 glass
1 kilogram (kg) or 1000 grams (Gm)	=	2.2 pounds (lb)

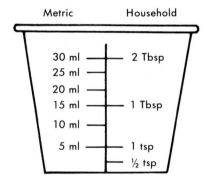

Conversion of measures between the metric and household systems of measure may also be done by the use of proportion, as has been illustrated.

EXAMPLE: 1½ c equals how many ml?

a. 1 c:180 ml::

b. 1 c:180ml:: _____ c: _____ ml

    1 c:180 ml:: 1½ c:x ml

c. 1:180::1 ½:x

d. $x = \dfrac{180}{1} \times \dfrac{3}{2}$

    $x = \dfrac{540}{2} = 270$ ml

e. 1 ½ c equals 270 ml

EXAMPLE: 35 kg equals how many pounds?

a. 1 kg:2.2 lb::

b. 1 kg:2.2 lb:: _____ kg: _____ lb

    1 kg:2.2 lb:: 35 kg: x lb.

c. 1:2.2::35:x

d. 1x = 2.2 × 35

    $x = 77$

e. 35 kg equals 77 lbs

Memorize the tables of the metric and household measurements. Study the material on forming proportions for the calculation of problems relating to the metric and household systems of measure. Complete the following work sheet, which provides for extensive practice in the manipulation of measurements within the metric and household systems. Check your answers. If you have difficulties, go back and review the necessary material. When you feel ready to evaluate your learning, take the first posttest. Check your answers. An acceptable score as indicated on the posttest signifies that you are ready for the next chapter. An unacceptable score signifies a need for further study before taking the second posttest.

WORK SHEET

Change to equivalents within the metric system. Solve the problems by the use of a
  proportion. Show your work.

1. 230 mcg = _____ Gm   **2.** 5 mg = _____ mcg   **3.** 2.5 Gm = _____ mcg

4. 4000 mcg = _____ mg   **5.** 0.33 Gm = _____ mg   **6.** 6 kg = _____ Gm

7. 725 ml = _____ L   **8.** 2000 mcg = _____ Gm   **9.** 0.75 L = _____ ml

10. 620 Gm = _____ kg   **11.** 36 cc = _____ ml   **12.** 460 ml = _____ L

13. 0.66 mg = _____ mcg   **14.** 0.5 Gm = _____ mcg   **15.** 474 L = _____ kl

16. 350,000 mcg = _____ Gm   **17.** 25 mg = _____ Gm   **18.** 1.46 L = _____ ml

19. 2.5 kg = _____ Gm   **20.** 12 mg = _____ mcg   **21.** 3.4 kg = _____ Gm

22. 920 mcg = _____ Gm   **23.** 250 Gm = _____ kg   **24.** 300 mcg = _____ mg

25. 0.16 L = _____ ml   **26.** 0.01 Gm = _____ mg   **27.** 500 mcg = _____ mg

28. 360 mg = _____ Gm

29. 3.25 kl = _____ L

30. 0.45 Gm = _____ mg

31. 240 ml = _____ L

32. 10 cc = _____ ml

Change the following household measurements into the approximate equivalents within the metric system. Solve the problems by the use of a proportion. Show your work.

33. 30 gtt = _____ ml

34. 1 ½ tsp = _____ ml

35. 2 ¼ c = _____ ml

36. 1 ⅖ Tbsp = _____ ml

37. 1 ⅓ glass = _____ ml

38. 4 Tbsp = _____ ml

39. ⅔ glass = _____ ml

40. 75 gtt = _____ ml

41. 1 ½ c = _____ ml

42. 3 tsp = _____ ml

43. 8 kg = _____ lb

44. 3825 Gm = _____ lb

45. 9 ½ lb = _____ Gm   **46.** 3 lb = _____ kg   **47.** 12 kg = _____ lb

48. 1400 Gm = _____ lb   **49.** 24 lb = _____ Gm   **50.** 150 lb = _____ kg

Answers on p. 355.

Name _____

Date _____

ACCEPTABLE SCORE ___27___

YOUR SCORE _____

POSTTEST 1

DIRECTIONS: Change to equivalent metric measurements. Solve each problem by the use of a
proportion. Show your work.

1. 5000 mcg = _____ Gm   **2.** 10 mg = _____ mcg   **3.** 0.81 L = _____ ml

4. 35 mg = _____ Gm   **5.** 1 ¾ tsp = _____ ml   **6.** 0.12 Gm = _____ mcg

7. 16 kg = _____ lb   **8.** 280 ml = _____ L   **9.** 0.4 kg = _____ Gm

10. 45 gtt = _____ ml   **11.** 28 lb = _____ Gm   **12.** 356 Gm = _____ kg

13. 500,000 mcg = _____ Gm

14. 37 ml = _____ L

15. 20 ml = _____ cc

16. 1 ⅕ c = _____ ml

17. 2.5 Gm = _____ mg

18. 12 cc = _____ ml

19. 6700 Gm = _____ kg

20. 0.3 kl = _____ L

21. 4 mg = _____ mcg

22. 2600 Gm = _____ lb

23. 1 ½ glass = _____ ml

24. 0.2 L = _____ ml

25. 533 L = _____ kl

26. 1.5 Gm = _____ mcg

27. 620 mg = _____ Gm

28. 2.3 kg = _____ Gm

29. 6 Tbsp = _____ ml

30. 7 lb = _____ kg

Answers on pp. 355-356.

Name _____

Date _____

ACCEPTABLE SCORE ___27___

YOUR SCORE _____

POSTTEST 2

DIRECTIONS: Change to equivalent metric measurements. Solve each problem by the use of a proportion. Show your work.

1. 4000 mcg = _____ mg

2. 150 Gm = _____ kg

3. 2 ½ c = _____ ml

4. 800 Gm = _____ lb

5. 44 kg = _____ lb

6. 760 mg = _____ Gm

7. 0.55 L = _____ ml

8. 788 L = _____ kl

9. ⅓ glass = _____ ml

10. 2 ⅛ lb = _____ Gm

11. 0.1 kl = _____ L

12. 32 mg = _____ mcg

13. 618 ml = _____ L

14. 100,000 mcg = _____ Gm

15. 90 gtt = _____ ml

16. 714 ml = _____ L

17. 350 L = _____ kl

18. 250,000 mcg = _____ Gm

19. 0.87 Gm = _____ mg

20. 7 mg = _____ mcg

21. 3 ¼ tsp = _____ ml

22. 1.4 kl = _____ L

23. 0.78 Gm = _____ mg

24. 225 mcg = _____ mg

25. 4500 Gm = _____ kg

26. 0.2 L = _____ ml

27. 2 Tbsp = _____ ml

28. 40 cc = _____ ml

29. 2.6 Gm = _____ mcg

30. 73 lb = _____ kg

Answers on p. 356.

Name _____

Date _____

ACCEPTABLE SCORE ___27___

YOUR SCORE _____

PRETEST

DIRECTIONS: Change to approximate equivalents as indicated. Solve the problem by the use of a proportion. Show your work.

1. 180 ♏ = _____ ml

2. 7 fl ʒ = _____ ml

3. 36 kg = _____ lb

4. 5 ¼ qt = _____ ml

5. 90 ml = _____ fl ʒ

6. 1 ¾ qt = _____ L

7. 90 gr = _____ Gm

8. 4.5 ml = _____ ♏

9. 8 ⅗ lb = _____ Gm

10. 2 ¼ pt = _____ ml

11. 7 fl ʒ = _____ ml

12. 10 gr = _____ Gm

13. 5.5 L = _____ qt

14. 5 ℳ = _____ ml

15. 4 gr = _____ mg

16. 360 ml = _____ fl ʒ

17. 600 ml = _____ pt

18. 5500 Gm = _____ lb

19. 20 ml = _____ fl ʒ

20. 12 mg = _____ gr

21. ⅟₃₀₀ gr = _____ mg

22. 85 lb = _____ kg

23. 0.4 mg = _____ gr

24. 2.4 ml = _____ ℳ

25. 4200 ml = _____ qt

26. 1 ½ fl ʒ = _____ ml

27. ⅕ gr = _____ mg

28. 4.6 Gm = _____ gr

29. 98.8° F = _____ °C

30. 41 °C = _____ °F

Answers on p. 356.

EQUIVALENTS BETWEEN APOTHECARIES' AND METRIC MEASUREMENTS

Learning objectives _____

On completion of the materials provided in this chapter, you will perform computations accurately by mastering the following mathematical concepts.

1. Recall equivalent apothecary and metric measures
2. Compute equivalents between the apothecaries' and metric systems by use of a proportion
3. Convert the Fahrenheit scale to the Celsius scale
4. Convert the Celsius scale to Fahrenheit scale

_____

One of a nurse's many responsibilities is the administration of medication. There are two different systems of measurements used in the calculation of drug dosages: the apothecaries' system and the metric system. Because hospitals and physicians use both systems, it is necessary for the nurse to be able to utilize both systems and know the approximate equivalents between the two systems.

Approximate equivalents between apothecaries' and metric measurements

A list of the most frequently used equivalents between apothecaries' and metric systems of measure is provided below. Memorize these equivalents.

Apothecaries' measures	Metric measures
15 minims (♏) =	1 milliliter (ml)
1 fluidram (fl ʒ) =	4 ml
1 fluidounce (fl ʒ) =	30 ml
6 fluidounces (fl ʒ) =	180 ml
8 fluidounces (fl ʒ) =	240 ml
16 fluidounces (fl ʒ) or 1 pint (pt) =	500 ml
32 fluidounces (fl ʒ) or 1 quart (qt) =	1000 ml or 1 liter (l)
1 grain (gr) =	60 milligrams (mg)
15 grains (gr) =	1 gram (Gm)
2.2 pounds (lb) =	1000 grams (Gm) or 1 kilogram (kg)

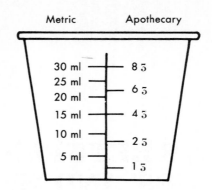

Sometimes the nurse will find it necessary to convert a medication order from one system to the other. This can be done by the use of a proportion.

EXAMPLE: 3 fl ʒ equals how many ml?

   a. On the left side of the proportion place what you know to be an equivalent between fluidrams and milliliters. In this example, the most appropriate equivalent is 1 fl ʒ = 4 ml. So the left side of the proportion would be

$$1 \text{ fl } ʒ : 4 \text{ ml.} : :$$

   b. The right side of the proportion will be determined by the problem and by the abbreviations used on the left side of the proportion. Only *two* different abbreviations may be used in a single proportion. The abbreviations must be in the same position on the right as they are on the left.

$$1 \text{ fl } ʒ : 4 \text{ ml} : : \underline{\hspace{2cm}} \text{ fl } ʒ : \underline{\hspace{2cm}} \text{ ml}$$

From the problem we know we have 3 fl ʒ.

$$1 \text{ fl } ʒ : 4 \text{ ml} : : 3 \text{ fl } ʒ : \underline{\hspace{2cm}} \text{ ml}$$

Since we need to find the number of milliliters in 3 fl ʒ, we use the symbol x to represent the unknown. Therefore the full proportion would be

$$1 \text{ fl } ʒ : 4 \text{ ml} : : 3 \text{ fl } ʒ : x \text{ ml}$$

   c. Rewrite the proportion without using the abbreviations.

$$1 : 4 : : 3 : x$$

   d. Solve for x.

$$1x = 4 \times 3$$
$$x = 12$$

   e. Label your answer, as determined by the abbreviation placed next to x in the original proportion.

$$3 \text{ fl } ʒ = 12 \text{ml}$$

EXAMPLE: 150 ml equals how many fl ʒ?

   a. 6 fl ʒ : 180 ml : :
   b. 6 fl ʒ : 180 ml : : \underline{\hspace{2cm}} fl ʒ : \underline{\hspace{2cm}} ml
      6 fl ʒ : 180 ml : : x fl ʒ : : 150 ml
   c. 6 : 180 : : x : 150

d. $180x = 900$

$$x = \frac{900}{180} = 5$$

e. 150 ml equals 5 fl ℥.

EXAMPLE: 45 mg equals how many grains?

a. 1 gr:60 mg::
b. 1 gr:60 mg:: _____ gr: _____ mg
   1 gr:60 mg::x gr:45 mg
c. 1:60::x:45
d. $60x = \dfrac{45}{60}$

   $x = \dfrac{3}{4}$
e. 45 mg equals ¾ gr

EXAMPLE: 18 ℳ equals how many milliliters?

a. 15 ℳ:1ml::
b. 15 ℳ:1 ml:: _____ ℳ: _____ ml
   15 ℳ:1 ml::18 ℳ:x ml
c. 15:1::18:x
d. $15x = 18$
   $x = 18 \div 15$
   $x = 1.2$
e. 18 ℳ equals 1.2 ml.

Approximate equivalents between Celsius and Fahrenheit measurements

Many hospitals and health care centers use the metric system of measurement, including thermometers calibrated in the Celsius scale. It may be necessary for the nurse to convert the Celsius, or centigrade, scale to the Fahrenheit scale for patient or family information. Since not everyone concerned with patient care uses one scale, it is also important for the nurse to be able to convert the Fahrenheit scale to the Celsius scale.

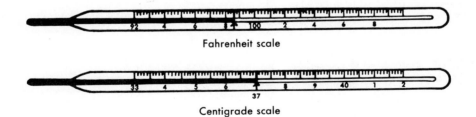

Fahrenheit scale

Centigrade scale

To convert one scale to another, use the following proportion:

Celsius:Fahrenheit − 32::5:9
C:F − 32::5:9

C or F will be the unknown.
Extend the decimal to hundredths, round to tenths.

EXAMPLE: 100.6° F equals _____ ° C.

C:F − 32::5:9

C:100.6 − 32::5:9

$$9C = (100.6 − 32) × 5$$
$$9C = 68.6 × 5$$
$$9C = 343$$
$$C = 343 ÷ 9$$
$$C = 38.11$$

100.6° F equals 38.1° C.

EXAMPLE: 37.6° C equals _____ ° F.

C:F − 32::5:9

37.6:F − 32::5:9
$$5 (F − 32) = 9 × 37.6$$
$$5F − 160 = 338.4$$

$$5F − 160 + 160 = 338.4 + 160$$

$$5F = 498.4$$
$$F = 498.4 ÷ 5$$
$$F = 99.68$$

37.8° C equals 99.7° F.

Memorize the table of approximate equivalents between apothecaries' and metric system of measure. Study the material on forming proportions for the calculations of problems converting between apothecaries' and metric systems of measure. Complete the following work sheet, which provides for extensive practice in the manipulation of measurements between apothecaries' and metric systems. Check your answers. If you have difficulties, go back and review the necessary material. When you feel ready to evaluate your learning, take the first posttest. Check your answers. An acceptable score as indicated on the posttest signifies that you are ready for the next chapter. An unacceptable score signifies a need for further study before taking the second posttest.

CHAPTER 8
EQUIVALENTS BETWEEN APOTHECARIES' AND METRIC MEASUREMENTS

WORK SHEET

Change to approximate equivalents as indicated. Solve the problems by the use of a
  proportion. Show your work.

1. 200 mg = _____ gr

2. 240 ℳ = _____ ml

3. 24 fl ʒ = _____ ml

4. 60 gr = _____ Gm

5. 300 ml = _____ fl ʒ

6. 150 gr = _____ Gm

7. 1¾ qt = _____ ml

8. 210 ml = _____ fl ℥

9. 40 ℳ = _____ ml

10. 10 kg = _____ lb

11. 1750 ml = _____ pt

12. ½ fl ℥ = _____ ml

13. 4 ½ gr = _____ mg

14. 4200 Gm = _____ lb

15. 420 mg = _____ gr

16. 5 ml = _____ ℳ

17. 6 pt = _____ ml

18. 3500 ml = _____ qt

19. 5 gr = _____ mg

20. 150 ml = _____ fl ℥

21. 30 ℳ = _____ ml

22. 6 fl ℥ = _____ ml

23. 3.3 Gm = _____ gr

24. 6 ⅘ lb = _____ Gm

25. 12 ml = _____ ℳ

26. ⅜ fl ℥ = _____ ml

27. 2 ¾ gr = _____ mg

28. 7 Gm = _____ gr

29. 5 lb = _____ kg

30. 2700 ml = _____ pt

31. 18 fl ℥ = _____ ml

32. 340 mg = _____ gr

33. 2 ½ qt = _____ L

34. 3650 Gm = _____ lb

35. 6000 ml = _____ qt

36. 8 fl ℥ = _____ ml

37. 8 ml = _____ ℳ

38. 45 gr = _____ Gm

39. 45 ℳ = _____ ml

40. 4 fl ℥ = _____ ml

41. 12 lb = _____ Gm

42. 75 ml = _____ fl ℥

43. 3 ml = _____ ℳ

44. 75 lb = _____ kg

45. 2 ⅛ qt = _____ ml

46. 100 mg = _____ gr

47. 3.5 L = _____ qt

48. 1½ gr = _____ mg

49. 3 pt = _____ ml

50. 25 kg = _____ lb

51. 99.6° F = _____ ° C

52. 101.8° F = _____ ° C

53. 104.2° F = _____ ° C.

54. 97.4° F = _____ ° C

55. 40.4° C = _____ ° F

56. 35.4° C = _____ ° F

57. 36.8° C = _____ ° F

58. 39.2° C = _____ ° F

Answers on p. 356.

Name _____

Date _____

ACCEPTABLE SCORE __27__

YOUR SCORE _____

POSTTEST 1

DIRECTIONS: Change to approximate equivalents as indicated. Solve the problem by the use of a proportion. Show your work.

1. 3 gr = _____ mg

2. 12 ♍ = _____ ml

3. 5 fl ℥ = _____ ml

4. 75 gr = _____ Gm

5. 3 fl ℥ = _____ ml

6. 1 ½ pt = _____ ml

7. 15 mg = _____ gr

8. 1500 ml = _____ qt

9. 7 ½ lb = _____ Gm

10. 260 ♍ = _____ ml

11. 1.7 L = _____ qt

12. 5 gr = _____ Gm

13. 8 ml = _____ fl ʒ

14. 20 lb = _____ kg

15. ⅙ gr = _____ mg

16. 1000 ml = _____ pt

17. 2 ml = _____ ♏

18. 0.3 mg = _____ gr

19. 3 Gm = _____ gr

20. 60 ml = _____ fl ʒ

21. 2700 Gm = _____ lb

22. 5 fl ʒ = _____ ml

23. 32 kg = _____ lb

24. 0.5 mg = _____ gr

25. 1.5 ml = _____ ♏

26. 80 gr = _____ Gm

27. 2 ¾ qt = _____ L

28. 540 ml = _____ fl ʒ

29. 95.4° F = _____ ° C

30. 35.6° C = _____ ° F.

Answers on p. 356.

170

Name _____

Date _____

ACCEPTABLE SCORE ___27___

YOUR SCORE _____

POSTTEST 2

DIRECTIONS: Change to approximate equivalents as indicated. Solve the problem by the use of proportion. Show your work.

1. 4.3 ml = _____ ℳ

2. 60 lb = _____ kg

3. 2500 ml = _____ qt

4. 4 gr = _____ Gm

5. 1 ¼ pt = _____ ml

6. ¼ gr = _____ mg

7. 1.25 L = _____ qt

8. 20 mg = _____ gr

9. 22 ½ ℳ = _____ ml

10. 20 lb = _____ Gm

11. ¾ pt = _____ ml

12. 2 ⅜ qt = _____ ml

13. 3 Gm = _____ gr

14. ¹/₁₂₀ gr = _____ mg

15. 10 fl ℥ = _____ ml

16. 7 gr = _____ Gm

17. 3 ½ qt = _____ L

18. 1500 ml = _____ pt

19. 1200 Gm = _____ lb

20. 10 ♏ = _____ ml

21. 0.8 mg = _____ gr

22. 42 kg = _____ lb

23. 12 fl ℥ = _____ ml

24. ¹/₂₀ gr = _____ mg

25. 1.4 ml = _____ ♏

26. 1.3 Gm = _____ gr

27. 3 ½ lb = _____ Gm

28. 10 ml = _____ fl ℥

29. 96.2° F = _____ ° C.

30. 38.2° C = _____ ° F

Answers on pp. 356-357.

PART III

Calculation of drug dosages

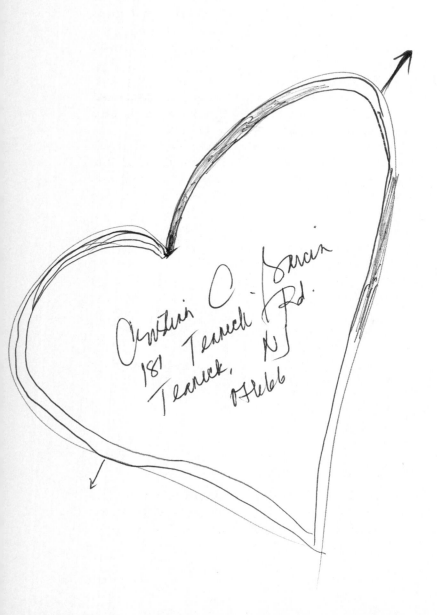

CHAPTER 9

INTERPRETATION OF THE PHYSICIAN'S ORDERS

Administration of medications is one of the most important responsibilities of the nurse. For medications to be administered safely and effectively, the nurse must know how to interpret the physician's medication orders.

Written orders

The physician prescribes the medications. In hospitals and health care centers, the physician uses a physician's order sheet, which is part of the patient's hospital chart or record. The orders are written for a drug to be given until a stated date and time, until a certain amount of the medication has been given, or until the order is changed or discontinued.

The physician's order requires the date the order was written, the name and dosage of the drug, the route and frequency of administration, and any special instructions. For drugs ordered as needed (p.r.n.), the purpose for administration is also added. The physician's signature is required each time orders are written.

To interpret the medication order, the nurse must know the terminology, abbreviations, and symbols used in writing medical prescriptions and orders for medications. A list of the most frequently used abbreviations and symbols relating to medications is listed in Table 1. Memorize this list. Refer to the Glossary for help with unfamiliar terms.

Verbal orders

While verbal orders are discouraged as routine policy, certain situations, usually emergencies may require telephone orders. Such orders are generally initiated by the nurse. The order must include the same information as the written order: the date the order is recorded, the name and dosage of the drug, the route and frequency of administration, and any special instructions. After the nurse has recorded the orders on the patient's chart, the orders must be repeated to the physician for verification. The physician's name, notation that this is a telephone order, and the nurse's signature are required. The physician should sign the verbal orders as soon as possible.

EXAMPLE

1/18/90 Demerol 100 mg I.M. q.4 h. p.r.n. for pain
     T.O. Dr. James T. Smith/Helen Alexander, R.N.

Scheduling the administration of medications

The physician's orders provide guidelines for the nurse when planning when each medication will be given to the patient. The purpose for prescribing the medication, drug interactions, absorption of the drug, or side effects caused by the drug may de-

Table 1. Recommended times for administering medications

Abbreviations	Definition	Recommended times of administration
a.c.*	before meals	7:30-11:30-5:30
a.m.	morning, before noon	9 a.m.
b.i.d.	twice a day	9-5
h.s.	at bedtime	9 p.m.
p.c.*	after meals	8:30-11:30-6:30
p.r.n.	as needed	
q.d.	once a day	10 a.m.
q.h.	every hour	8-9-10-etc.
q 2h.	every 2 hours	8-10-12-etc.
q 3h.	every 3 hours	9-12-3-etc.
q 4h.	every 4 hours	8-12-4-etc.
q 6h.	every 6 hours	9-3-9-3
q 8h.	every 8 hours	8-4-12
q 12h.	every 12 hours	8-8
q.i.d.	four times a day	8-12-4-8
q.o.d.	every other day	
q.o.h.	every other hour	8-10-12-2-4-6-etc.
s.o.s.	once if necessary	
STAT	immediately	
t.i.d.	three times a day	9-1-5

*Providing meals are served at 8:00 a.m., 12:00 noon, and 6:00 p.m.

Table 2. Conversion from military time to a.m.-p.m. time

0100 — 1:00 a.m.	0900 — 9:00 a.m.	1700 — 5:00 p.m.
0200 — 2:00 a.m.	1000 — 10:00 a.m.	1800 — 6:00 p.m.
0300 — 3:00 a.m.	1100 — 11:00 a.m.	1900 — 7:00 p.m.
0400 — 4:00 a.m.	1200 — 12:00 noon	2000 — 8:00 p.m.
0500 — 5:00 a.m.	1300 — 1:00 p.m.	2100 — 9:00 p.m.
0600 — 6:00 a.m.	1400 — 2:00 p.m.	2200 — 10:00 p.m.
0700 — 7:00 a.m.	1500 — 3:00 p.m.	2300 — 11:00 p.m.
0800 — 8:00 a.m.	1600 — 4:00 p.m.	2400 — 12:00 midnight

termine when the drug is given. The prescribed order may be very specific or may give the nurse latitude in scheduling.

Most hospitals and health care centers have routine times for administering medications. These time may differ from one hospital to another, but the guidelines assist the nurse to plan a medication routine that is safe for the patient. Table 1 will assist in planning times for administering each medication. Many hospitals are using military time rather than ante meridian (a.m.) and post meridian (p.m.) time. Table 2 will assist in conversion from military time. Military time can be quickly computed by adding 12 to p.m. time—for example, 12 + 3 = 1500 hours.

Introduction to drug dosages

The nurse obtains the medication from the pharmacy or from an available supply on the clinical unit, prepares the dosage, and administers the medication. Unit dosages are prepared in individual doses by the manufacturer and are ready for the nurse to administer.

Most medications are secured in the required dosage. However, problems of drug calculation arise when a drug is not manufactured in the strength required by the patient, the drug is not available in the strength ordered, or the drug is ordered in one system of measurement but is available only in another system of measurement.

When you change from one system of measurement to another, you have an equivalent measure that may or may not be exact. Therefore, the answer to your problem may vary according to the system of measurement used. For example, if you change the required dosage to the available dosage, the equivalent dosage may be different than if you changed to the available dosage to the required dosage. All problems in this book are calculated by changing the required dosage to the available dosage. The answers reflect this method of calculation. This is good practice because you have the medication at hand in the dosage provided.

The remainder of this book is devoted to problems relating to the calculation of various types of dosage problems. The nurse is responsible for giving the right amount of the right medication to the right patient at the right time and in the right way. The nurse is ethically and legally responsible for the medications administered to the patient. Even though the physician writes the order for the medication to be given to the patient or even if the pharmacy prepares the wrong medication, the nurse who administers the medication is responsible for the error. Before preparing the drug, the nurse *must know* the maximum and minimum dosages and the actions and contraindications for each administered drug. In addition, the nurse should consult the patient for any known allergies.

The nurse must also have the mathematical skills required to calculate drug dosage problems. It is absolutely essential that the dosages be calculated accurately. If a nurse has any doubts concerning the dosages, another nurse should be consulted.

Most problems relating to drug dosages in this workbook can be solved by the use of a proportion. If you have mastered the material presented in this workbook thus far, you are prepared to study the various types of problems in the following chapters relating to drug dosage.

PRETEST

DIRECTIONS: The medication order is listed at the beginning of each problem. Calculate the oral dosages by the use of proportions. Show your work. Place your answer in the space provided and label.

1. Enduron 2.5 mg p.o. q.d. You have Enduron 5 mg grooved tablet. Give _____ .

2. Vistaril gr. i p.o. q.6h. Vistaril Oral Suspension 25 mg per 5 ml is supplied. Give _____ .

3. Glipizide 10 mg p.o. q. A.M. The drug is supplied in 5 mg. scored tablets. Give _____ .

4. Tagamet 400 mg p.o. h.s. Tagamet is supplied 300 mg per ml. Give _____ .

5. Phenobarbital 0.06 Gm p.o. p.r.n. Phenobarbital elixir gr s̄s̄ per 7.5 ml is available. Give _____ .

6. Crystodigin gr. 1/300 p.o.q.i.d. You have 0.1 mg tablets available. Give _____ .

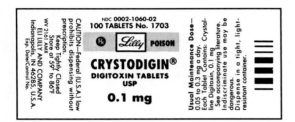

7. Demerol 0.025 Gm. p.o. q.4h. p.r.n. Demerol 50 mg tablets are available. Give _____ .

8. Codeine gr. 1/2 p.o. q.3h. p.r.n. You have codeine tablets gr 1/4 available. Give _____ .

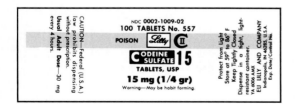

9. Thorazine 25 mg p.o. t.i.d. Thorazine Syrup is supplied in ℥ iv bottles containing 10 mg per 5 ml. Give _____ .

10. Gantrisin 1 Gm. p.o. q.6h. You have tablets gr viiss available. Give _____ .

11. Ampicillin 0.2 Gm p.o. q.6 h. Ampicillin Oral Suspension 125 mg per 5 ml is available. Give _____ .

12. Lanoxin 0.125 mg p.o. q.i.d. You have 0.25 mg tablets available. Give _____ .

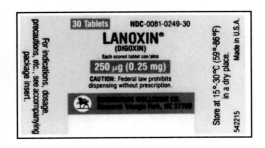

13. Orinase 750 mg p.o. b.i.d. You have 0.5 Gm tablets available. Give _____ .

14. Dicumarol 200 mg p.o. stat. Dicumarol 50 mg tablets are available. Give _____ .

15. Acetaminophen gr x p.o. q. 4h. The drug is supplied in 325 mg tablets. Give _____ .

16. Seconal 200 mg p.o. h.s. You have 100 mg capsules available. Give _____ .

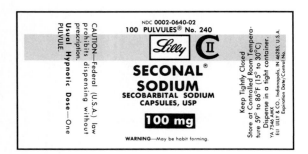

17. A.S.A. 600 mg p.o. q.3h. p.r.n. You have gr v tablets available. Give _____ .

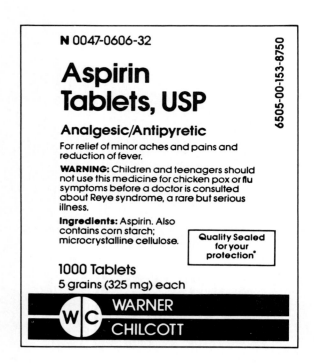

18. KCl 10 mEq p.o. b.i.d. KCl liquid 20 mEq per 30 ml is available. Give _____ .

19. Keflex 0.5 Gm p.o. q.i.d. You have Keflex capsules 250 mg available. Give _____ .

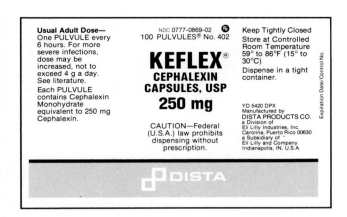

20. Elixir of Benadryl ʒ ii p.o. t.i.d. You have a ʒ xvi bottle containing 12.5 mg per ʒ. How many mg will you give for each dose? _____ .
How many doses will each bottle provide? _____ .

Answers on p. 357.

CHAPTER 10
ORAL DOSAGES

Learning objectives

On completion of the materials provided in this chapter, you will be able to perform computations accurately by mastering the following mathematical concepts:

1. Convert all measures within the problem to equivalent measures in one system of measurement
2. Use a proportion to solve problems of oral dosage involving tablets, capsules, or liquid medications.
3. Use a proportion to solve problems of oral dosages of medications measured in milliequivalents

Oral drugs are the method of choice for administration of medications because they are easy to take and convenient for the patient. They are safe because they can be taken through the gastrointestinal tract, so that the skin is not interrupted. Oral medications may be more economical, since the production cost is usually lower than that for other forms of medications.

Oral medications are absorbed primarily in the small intestines. Because of the differences in absorption factors they might not be as effective as other forms of medications. Some oral medications are irritating to the alimentary canal and must be given with meals or a snack. Others may be harmful to the teeth and should be taken through a straw or feeding tube.

The most common types of oral medications are liquids, tablets, capsules, and caplets. Grooved or scored tablets may be divided, so that one half or one fourth of a tablet may be used.

Oral dosages involving capsules and tablets

EXAMPLE: A.S.A. gr. xx p.o. q.i.d. A.S.A. tablets gr. v are available. Give _____ .

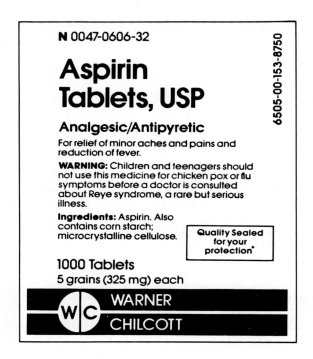

a. On the left side of the proportion place what you know or have available. In this example, each tablet equals 5 grains. So the left side of the proportion would be

$$1 \text{ tablet} : 5 \text{ gr} : :$$

b. The right side of the proportion is determined by the physician's order and the abbreviations used on the left side of the proportion. Only *two* different abbreviations may be used in a single proportion. The abbreviations must be in the same position on the right as they are on the left.

$$1 \text{ tablet} : 5 \text{ gr} : : \text{_____ tablet} : \text{_____ gr}$$

In the example the physician has ordered 20 grains.

$$1 \text{ tablet} : 5 \text{ gr} : : \text{_____ tablet} : 20 \text{ gr}$$

Since we need to find the number of tablets to be given, we use the symbol x to represent the unknown. Therefore the full proportion would be

$$1 \text{ tablet} : 5 \text{ gr} : : x \text{ tablet} : 20 \text{ gr}$$

c. Rewrite the proportion without using the abbreviations.

$$1 : 5 : : x : 20$$

d. Solve for x.

$$5x = 1 \times 20$$

$$5x = 20$$

$$x = \frac{20}{5}$$

$$x = 4$$

e. Label your answer, as determined by the abbreviation placed next to x in the original proportion.

$$20 \text{ gr} = 4 \text{ tablets}$$

Sometimes the physician's order is in one system of measurement, and the drug is supplied in another system of measurement. It is therefore necessary to convert one of the measurements so that they are both in either the apothecaries' or the metric system of measurement. After this is done, another proportion will be set up to calculate the actual drug dosage.

EXAMPLE: Ampicillin 0.5 Gm p.o. q.i.d. The drug is supplied in 250 mg capsules.

Give _____ .

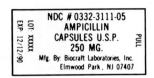

The physician's order is in grams and the drug is supplied in milligrams. It is necessary for the order and the supplied drug to be in the same metric measurement, since only two different abbreviations can be used in each proportion. Therefore, either convert 0.5 Gm to milligrams or convert 250 mg to grains, whichever you prefer.

$$1000 \text{ mg} : 1 \text{ Gm} :: x \text{ mg} : 0.5 \text{ Gm}$$

$$1000 : 1 :: x : 0.5$$

$$1x = 1000 \times 0.5$$

$$x = 500 \text{ mg}$$

Now that the order and the supplied drug are in the same metric measurement, a proportion may be written to calculate the amount of the drug to be given.

a. 250 mg : 1 capsule ::

b. 250 mg : 1 capsule :: _____ mg : _____ capsule

250 mg : 1 capsule :: 500 mg : x capsule

c. 250 : 1 :: 500 : x

d. $250x = 1 \times 500$

$250x = 500$

$$x = \frac{500}{250}$$

$x = 2$

e. $x = 2$ capsules. Therefore, 2 capsules, or 0.5 Gm, of the medication ordered would be given to the patient.

How many capsules will be given in one day? _____

The drug is to be given q.i.d., or four times a day.

a. 2 capsules : 1 dose ::

b. 2 capsules : 1 dose :: _____ capsules : _____ dose

2 capsules : 1 dose :: x capsules : 4 doses

c. 2 : 1 :: x : 4

d. $1x = 2 \times 4$

$x = 8$

e. 8 capsules will given each day.

Oral dosages involving liquids

EXAMPLE: Phenobarbital gr ¾ p.o. b.i.d. Phenobarbital elixir 20 mg per 5 ml is available. Give _____ . The physician's order is in the apothecaries' system and the drug is available in the metric system. It is first necessary for both the order and the available drug to be in the same system of measurement. Therefore either convert gr ¾ to milligrams or convert 20 mg to grains, whichever you prefer.

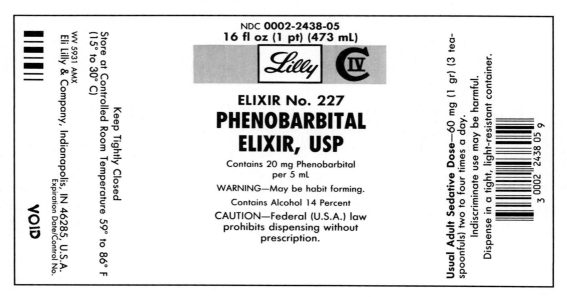

$$60 \text{ mg} : 1 \text{ gr} : : x \text{ mg} : \frac{3}{4} \text{ gr}$$

$$60 : 1 : : x : \frac{3}{4}$$

$$x = \frac{\overset{15}{\cancel{60}}}{1} \times \frac{3}{\underset{1}{\cancel{4}}}$$

$$x = 45 \text{ mg}$$

$$\text{gr} \frac{3}{4} = 45 \text{ mg}$$

Now that the order and available drug are in the same system of measurement, a proportion may be written to calculate the actual amount of the drug to be administered.

   a. 20 mg:5 ml ::

   b. 20 mg :5 ml :: _____ mg : _____ ml

      20 mg :5 ml ::45 mg :x ml

   c. 20:5 ::45:x

   d. $20x = 5 \times 45$

      $20x = 225$

      $x = \dfrac{225}{20}$

      $x = 11.25$

   e. $x = 11.25$ ml. Therefore 11.25 ml is the amount of each individual dose b.i.d.

EXAMPLE: Thorazine 20 mg p.o. q.4.h. The drug is available in ℥ iv bottles of Thorazine Syrup containing 10 mg per 5 ml. Give _____ . How many doses are available in ℥ iv? _____ .

1. a. 10 mg : 5 ml : :
    b. 10 mg : 5 ml : : _____ mg: _____ ml
       10 mg : 5 ml : : 20 mg : x ml
    c. 10:5::20:x
    d. $10x = 5 \times 20$

       $10x = 100$

       $x = \dfrac{100}{10}$

       $x = 10$
    e. $x = 10$ ml. Therefore 10 ml is the amount of each individual dose q.4 h.

2. The physician's order is in the metric system and the drug is supplied in the apothecaries' system. It is necessary for both the order and the available drug to be in the same system of measurement. Therefore, convert 10 ml to ℥ or the ℥ iv to ml whichever is easier.

    $$30 \text{ ml}: 1 \text{ fl℥}::x \text{ ml}: 4 \text{ fl℥}$$

    $$30:1::x:4$$

    $$x = 120$$

    $$℥ \text{ iv bottle} = 120 \text{ ml}$$

    Now that the order and available drug are in the same system of measurement, a proportion may be written to calculate the number of doses in ℥ iv bottle.

    a. 10 ml: 1 dose : :
    b. 10 ml: 1 dose : : _____ ml: _____ dose
       10 ml : 1 dose : : 120 ml : x dose
    c. 10: 1 : : 120:x
    d. $10x = 120$

       $x = \dfrac{120}{10}$

       $x = 12$
    e. $x = 12$ doses. Therefore each ℥ iv bottle contains 12 doses.

Oral dosages involving milliequivalents

EXAMPLE: : KC1 60 mEq. KC1 40 mEq per 30 ml is available. Give _____ .

A milliequivalent is defined as the number of grams of a solute contained in one milliliter of a normal solution. The milliequivalent is utilized in a drug dosage proportion, the same as with a form of measurement in the apothecary or metric systems.

    a. 40 mEq : 30 ml : :
    b. 40 mEq : 30 ml : : _____ mEq : _____ ml
       40 mEq : 30 ml : : 60 mEq : x ml
    c. 40 : 30 : : 60 : x

d. $40x = 30 \times 60$
   $40x = 1800$

   $$x = \frac{1800}{40}$$

   $x = 45$

e. $x = 45$ ml

Complete the following work sheet, which provides for extensive practice in the calculation of oral dosage problems. Check your answers. It is sometimes impossible to administer the exact amount ordered. All capsules and those tablets not grooved are impossible to divide accurately. If the exact answer contains a fraction less than one half, drop the fraction and give the number of capsules or tablets indicated by the whole number. If the fraction is one half or more, round off to the nearest whole number to determine the number of tablets or capsules to be given. If you have difficulties, go back and review the necessary material. When you feel ready to evaluate your learning, take the first posttest. Check your answers. An acceptable score as indicated on the posttest signifies that you are ready for the next chapter. An unacceptable score signifies a need for further study before taking the second posttest.

WORK SHEET

The medication order is listed at the beginning of each problem. Calculate the oral dosages by the use of a proportion. Show your work. Place your answers in the space provided and label.

1. Minipress 2 mg p.o. b.i.d. Mini-press 1 mg capsules are available. Give _____ .

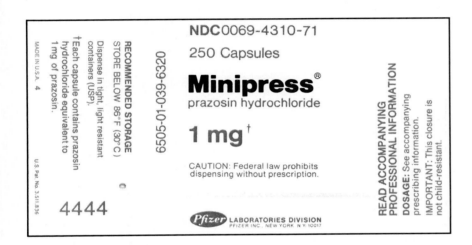

2. Elixir of phenobarbital 30 mg p.o. q. 12 h. The stock supply is elixir of phenobarbital 20 mg. per 5 ml. Give _____ .

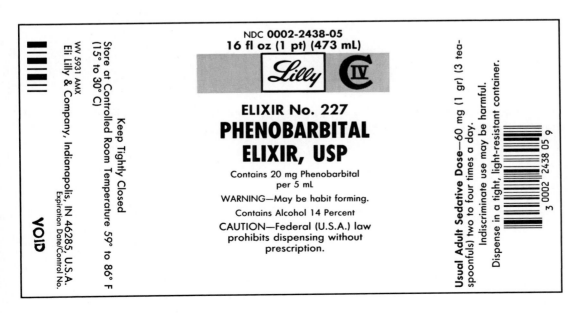

3. Crystodigin 0.2 mg p.o. b.i.d. for 4 days, then 0.15 mg q.d. You have Crystodigin 0.05 mg tablets available. How many tablets would you give for each dose the first four days? _____ . How many tablets would be given for each dose thereafter? _____ .

4. Thorazine gr ⅙ p.o. q. 8 h. for nausea. The drug is available in 10 mg tablets. Give _____ .

100 tablets **10**mg.
NDC 0007-5073-21

Thorazine®
brand of
chlorpromazine HCl
Tablets

Each tablet contains chlorpromazine hydrochloride, 10 mg.
Dosage: See package insert for dosage information.

STORE AT CONTROLLED
ROOM TEMPERATURE

Smith Kline &French Laboratories
Div. of SmithKline Beckman Corporation
Philadelphia, Pa. 19101

SK&F

5. Compazine 2.5 mg. p.o. t.i.d. The stock supply is Compazine Syrup 5 mg per 5 ml. Give _____ .

6. Temaril 2.5 mg p.o. q. 4h. The drug is supplied in ℥ iv bottles containing 2.5 mg per 5 ml. How many doses are available in ℥ iv? _____ .

7. Librium 10 mg p.o. q.6 h. You have Librium capsules gr ¹⁄₁₂. Give _____ .

8. Mandelamine 1 Gm p.o. q.i.d. You have 0.5 Gm tablets available. Give _____ .

9. Noctec 0.5 Gm p.o. h.s. p.r.n. The drug is available as 500 mg per ℥. Hom many ml will you give? _____ .

10. Cogentin 1 mg p.o. 7:00 P.M. The drug is available in 0.5 mg tablets. Give _____ .

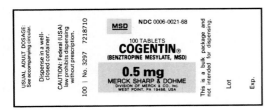

11. Motrin 300 mg p.o. t.i.d. The drug is supplied in gr v tablets. Give _____ .

12. Lithium carbonate 0.6 Gm p.o. b.i.d. The drug is supplied in 300 mg scored tablets. Give _____ . How many mg will be given each day? _____ .

13. Naprosyn 0.25 Gm p.o. b.i.d. You have Naprosyn 500 mg scored tablets. Give _____ .

14. Persantine 25 mg p.o. b.i.d. Persantine 50 mg tablets are available. Give _____ .

15. FeSO$_4$ 300 mg p.o. q.d. You have FeSo$_4$ gr v tablets available. Give _____ .

NDC 0002-0313-02
100 TABLETS No. 1571

Lilly

FERROUS SULFATE TABLETS USP

5 grs (324 mg)

For Iron Deficiency in Hypochromic Anemias.

Do not purchase if Lilly band around cap is missing or broken. After purchasing, do not use initially if red Lilly seal under cap is missing or broken. Tampering may have occurred.

Usual Adult Dose—One or two tablets 3 times a day after meals, or as directed by the physician. Infants and children only as directed by the physician since indiscriminate use or large doses may be harmful to them. **WARNINGS: Keep all medications out of the reach of children.** As with any drug, if you are pregnant or nursing a baby, seek the advice of a health professional before using this product.

Each Tablet equivalent to 65 mg elemental iron. Also contains cellulose, F D & C Blue No. 1, F D & C Red No. 40, F D & C Yellow No. 6, lactose, magnesium stearate, silicon dioxide, sodium lauryl sulfate, talc, titanium dioxide and other inactive ingredients.
Keep Tightly Closed
Store at 59° to 86°F
YA-8009 AMX
Eli Lilly & Co., Indianapolis, IN 46285, U.S.A.
Expiration Date/Control No.

$$\frac{300}{324} \longrightarrow \quad 300 \overline{)300}$$

$$\frac{60}{\frac{5}{300}}$$

$$\boxed{1\,tab}$$

16. Gantrisin 4 Gm p.o. stat., then 2 Gm q. 6 h. Gantrisin is supplied in 0.5 Gm tablets. How many tablets are given for the stat. dose? _____ . How many tablets are given for each of the 2 Gm doses? _____ .

17. Chloral hydrate 90 mg p.o. stat. Chloral hydrate 500 mg per 10 ml is available. Give _____ .

18. Gaviscon 30 ml p.o. q.i.d. p.c. h.s. Gaviscon is supplied in ℥ xii bottles. Each dose is equal to _____ ℥. How many would be given in one day? _____ .

19. Benadryl 30 mg p.o. t.i.d. You have Elixir of Benadryl 12.5 mg per 5 ml. Give _____ .

20. Codeine 60 mg p.o. q. 3 h. p.r.n. You have gr ¼ tablets. Give _____ .

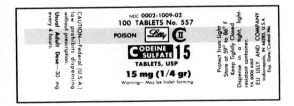

21. Keflex Suspension 5.5 ml p.o. q. 6 h. You have 125 mg per 5 ml. How many mg will you give q. 6 h.? _____ .

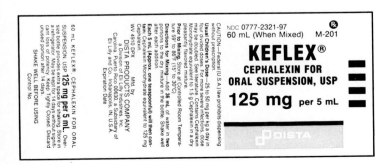

22. Lasix 80 mg p.o. q.d. You have Lasix 40 mg tablets available. Give _____ .

```
┌─────────────────────────────────────────────────────────────────┐
│ Keep this and all medi-   NDC 0039-0060-10   Usual Dosage: 20 to  │
│ cation out of the reach                      80 mg. See insert for│
│ of children.              Lasix®             full prescribing     │
│ Store at room tem-                           information.         │
│ perature.                 (furosemide)       Dispense in well-    │
│ NSN 6505-00-082-3336                         closed,              │
│ Lasix REG TM HOECHST AG   40 mg              light-resistant      │
│                                              containers           │
│ ℞ REG TM HOECHST AG                          with safety closures.│
│ HOECHST-ROUSSEL          Caution: Federal law prohibits  Lot:     │
│ Pharmaceuticals Inc.     dispensing without prescription. Exp:    │
│ Somerville, N.J. 08876   100 Tablets  40 mg                       │
│ 660100-2/87                                                       │
└─────────────────────────────────────────────────────────────────┘
```

23. Achromycin-V 0.5 Gm p.o. q.i.d. The drug is available in 250 mg capsules. How many capsules will you give for one dose? _____ . How many capsules will the patient receive in one day? _____ .

24. Decadron 1.5 mg p.o. q. 12 h. You have Decadron Elixir 0.5 mg per 5 ml. How many ml would you give? _____ How many ℥ would you give? _____ .

25. Thorazine 15 mg p.o. q. 4 h. The drug is available in ℥ iv bottles of Thorazine Syrup containing 10 mg per 5 ml. Give _____ .

26. Apresoline 25 mg p.o. q.i.d. You have available 50 mg tablets. Give _____ .

27. Mylanta 30 ml p.o. p.c. q.i.d. Mylanta is supplied in a ʒ xii bottle. How many doses does one ʒ xii bottle provide? _____ .

28. Thorazine 30 mg p.o. t.i.d. The drug is available in Thorazine Syrup 10 mg per ʒ. Give _____ .

29. Phenobarbital 15 mg p.o. q. 3 h. You have phenobarbital tablets gr ½. Give _____ .

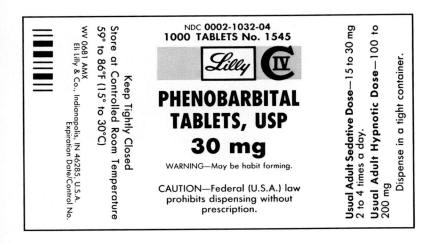

30. Amoxil 250 mg p.o. q. 8 h. The drug is available in a 150 ml bottle containing 125 mg per 5 ml. Give _____ .

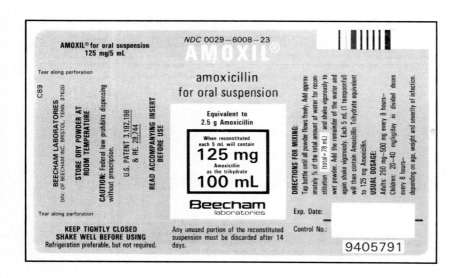

31. Tenormin 25 mg p.o. q. 4 h. You have Tenormin 50 mg scored tablets. Give _____ .

32. Quinidine 0.6 Gm p.o. q. 4 h. Quinidine is supplied in 200 mg tablets. How many tablets would you give for one dose? _____ . How many tablets will be given in 24 hours? _____ .

33. Phenergan 12.5 mg p.o. t.i.d. The drug is available in syrup containing 6.25 mg per 3. Give _____ .

34. Dalmane 30 mg p.o. h.s. You have Dalmane capsules gr ¼. Give _____ .

35. Colace Elixir 100 mg p.o. h.s. You have Colace 20 mg per 5 ml. Give _____ .

NDC 0087-0720-01

SYRUP

COLACE®

DOCUSATE SODIUM

STOOL SOFTENER

8 FL OZ (½ PT)

MeadJohnson

Do not use if carton overwrap was missing or broken.

COLACE is used for prevention of dry, hard stools.

Usual daily dose

Infants and children under 3: As prescribed by physician.

Children 3 to 6: 1 to 3 teaspoons.

Children 6 to 12: 2 teaspoons one to three times daily.

Adults and older children: 1 to 3 tablespoons.

Keep this and all medication out of reach of children.

•P7169-09
•P7169-09
•P7169-09

The effect of COLACE on the stools may not be apparent until 1 to 3 days after first oral dose.

WARNING: As with any drug, if you are pregnant or nursing a baby, seek the advice of a health professional before using this product.

Each teaspoon (5 ml) contains 20 mg docusate sodium; each tablespoon (15 ml) contains 60 mg. Contains not more than 1% alcohol.

Store at room temperature. Protect from excessive heat.

MEAD JOHNSON PHARMACEUTICALS
Bristol-Myers
U.S. Pharmaceutical and Nutritional Group
Evansville, IN 47721
Made in U.S.A.

36. KC1 80 mEq p.o. q.d. You have a liquid containing 40 mEq per 30 ml. Give _____ .

37. Deltasone 7.5 mg p.o. t.i.d. The drug is available in 2.5 mg tablets. Give _____ .

38. Tegretol 0.2 Gm p.o. t.i.d. You have Tegretol tablets 100 mg. Give _____ . How many mg will be given each day? _____ .

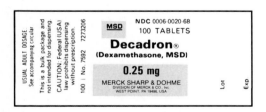

39. Elixir of Tylenol gr v p.o. t.i.d. You have the drug containing 160 mg per 5 ml. Give _____ .

40. Decadron 0.5 mg p.o. q. 12 h. You have 0.25 mg tablets. Give _____ .

41. Compazine 10 mg p.o. q. 4 h. p.r.n. You have Compazine 5 mg tablets. Give _____ .

42. Atarax 100 mg p.o. h.s. p.r.n. You have 50 mg tablets available. Give _____ .

43. Thyroid gr ss p.o. q.i.d. Thyroid tablets 30 mg are available. Give _____ .

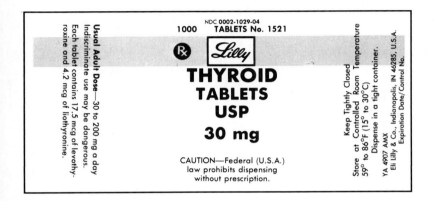

44. Lanoxin 0.25 mg p.o. q.d. The drug is supplied in 0.125 mg tablets. Give _____ .

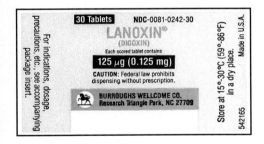

45. Keflex 500 mg p.o. q.i.d. You have 250 mg capsules available. How many capsules will you give for one dose? _____ . How many capsules will you give in one day? _____ .

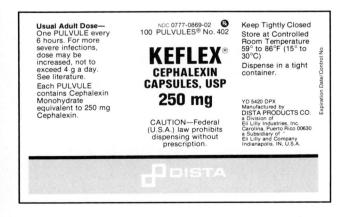

46. Valium 5 mg p.o. q. 6 h. p.r.n. You have 10 mg tablets. Give _____ .

47. Phenobarbital tablets gr i ss p.o. q. 3 h. p.r.n. The drug is supplied in 30 mg tablets. Give _____ .

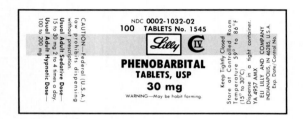

48. KCl 2 mEq p.o. q. 8 h. KCl 15 mEq per 11.25 ml is available. Give _____ .

49. A.S.A. gr x p.o. q. 3 h. You have A.S.A. 0.3 Gm tablets. Give _____ .

50. Terpin hydrate 10 ml p.o. q. 4h. p.r.n. Give _____ ʒ.

51. Erythromycin 1 Gm p.o. q. 6 h. You have 250 mg capsules. Give _____ .

52. FeSO$_4$ gr v p.o. t.i.d. You have 0.3 Gm tablets available. Give _____ .

```
        NDC 0002-0313-02
        100 TABLETS No. 1571
              Lilly
        FERROUS
        SULFATE
        TABLETS
        USP
        5 grs (324 mg)
        For Iron Deficiency in
        Hypochromic Anemias.
```

53. Bentyl 20 mg p.o. t.i.d. a.c. The drug is available in 10 mg capsules. Give _____ .

54. Atarax 30 mg p.o. b.i.d. The drug is supplied in syrup containing 10 mg per teaspoon. Give _____ .

55. Ascorbic acid 0.75 Gm p.o. daily. You have 250 mg tablets available. Give _____ .

56. Phenergan 25 mg p.o. q. 4 h. p.r.n. The drug is supplied in 12.5 mg tablets. Give _____ .

57. Vistaril 15 mg p.o. q.i.d. You have Vistaril 25 mg per 5 ml. Give _____ .

58. Terramycin 1.5 Gm p.o. stat.; then give 0.5 Gm q.i.d. until a total of 9 Gm is given. Terramycin is supplied in 250 mg capsules. How many capsules will be given stat.? _____ . How many capsules will be given for each q.i.d. dose? _____ . How many capsules will be given in one day when given q.i.d.? _____ . How many doses in addition to the stat. dose will be required to give 9 Gm of the drug? _____ .

59. Noctec Elixir 250 mg p.o. q. h.s. p.r.n. You have 500 mg per 5 ml. Give _____ .

60. Chloromycetin 250 mg p.o. q. 6 h. You have Chloromycetin 150 mg per 5 ml. Give _____ .

61. Vibramycin 100 mg p.o. q. 12 h. The drug is supplied 50 mg per 5 ml. How many ml will you give? _____ .

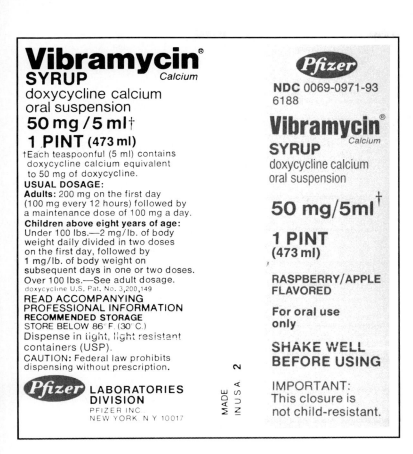

Vibramycin®
SYRUP   *Calcium*
doxycycline calcium
oral suspension
50 mg / 5 ml†
1 PINT (473 ml)
†Each teaspoonful (5 ml) contains
doxycycline calcium equivalent
to 50 mg of doxycycline.
USUAL DOSAGE:
Adults: 200 mg on the first day
(100 mg every 12 hours) followed by
a maintenance dose of 100 mg a day.
Children above eight years of age:
Under 100 lbs.—2 mg/lb. of body
weight daily divided in two doses
on the first day, followed by
1 mg/lb. of body weight on
subsequent days in one or two doses.
Over 100 lbs.—See adult dosage.
doxycycline U.S. Pat. No. 3,200,149
READ ACCOMPANYING
PROFESSIONAL INFORMATION
RECOMMENDED STORAGE
STORE BELOW 86° F. (30° C.)
Dispense in tight, light resistant
containers (USP).
CAUTION: Federal law prohibits
dispensing without prescription.

Pfizer **LABORATORIES
DIVISION**
PFIZER INC
NEW YORK N Y 10017

MADE
IN U S A 2

Pfizer
NDC 0069-0971-93
6188
Vibramycin®
Calcium
SYRUP
doxycycline calcium
oral suspension

50 mg/5ml†

1 PINT
(473 ml)

RASPBERRY/APPLE
FLAVORED

**For oral use
only**

**SHAKE WELL
BEFORE USING**

IMPORTANT:
This closure is
not child-resistant.

62. HydroDiuril 25 mg p.o. b.i.d. You have 50 mg tablets. Give _____ .

63. Tylenol 240 mg p.o. q. 4 h. for temperature 38.9° C. You have Tylenol 80 mg chewable tablets available. How many tablets will be required for each dose? _____ .

64. Lanoxin elixir 90 mcg p.o. b.i.d. from a stock supply containing 0.05 mg per ml. Give _____ .

65. Elixir of Benadryl, 10 ml p.o. q. 6 h. p.r.n. The drug is supplied 12.5 mg per ml. How many mg will you give? _____ .

66. Orinase 0.5 Gm p.o. t.i.d. Orinase 500 mg tablets are available. Give _____ .

67. Dilantin gr. iss p.o. t.i.d. You have 30 mg capsules. Give _____ .

68. Milk of Magnesia 2 Tbsp p.o. h.s. Give _____ ℥, or _____ ℨ.

69. KC1 10 mEq p.o. q.d. The drug is available in liquid, 20 mEq per 15 ml. Give _____ .

70. Nalfon 300 mg p.o. c̄ meals or a snack. Nalfon is supplied in 600 mg scored tablets. Give _____ .

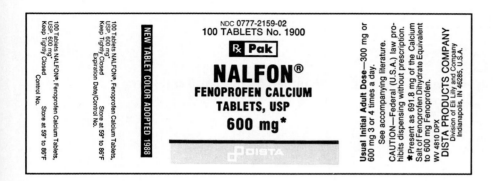

71. Digoxin 0.5 mg p.o. q.d. The drug is available in 0.25 mg tablets. Give _____ .

72. Tylenol 650 mg p.o. q. 4 h. for temperature of more than 38.5° C × 24 h. Extra-Strength Tylenol adult liquid 1000 mg per 30 ml is available. Give _____ ml q. 4 h.

73. Decadron 0.5 mg p.o. q. 12 h. You have 0.25 mg tablets. Give _____ .

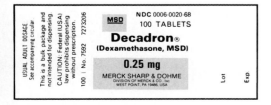

74. Keflex ℥ ss p.o. q. 6 h. Keflex Oral Suspension is supplied as 125 mg per 5 ml. How many mg will be given? _____ .

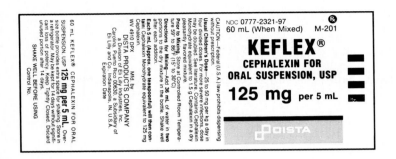

75. Demerol 30 mg p.o. q. 4 h. p.r.n. The drug is supplied 50 mg per 5 ml. Give _____ .

76. Crystodigin gr ½₀₀ p.o. q.d. You have Crystodigin in 0.05, 0.15, and 0.2 mg tablets. Give _____ tablets of _____ mg.

77. Prednisone 7.5 mg p.o. q.d. Prednisone is supplied in 5 mg grooved tablets. Give _____ .

78. V-Cillin K Suspension 250 mg p.o. q.i.d. The drug is supplied 125 mg. per 5 ml. Give
_____ .

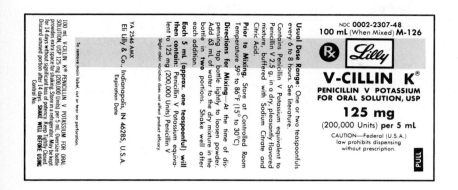

79. Surfak 250 mg p.o. q.d. Surfak is supplied in 50 mg capsules. Give _____ .

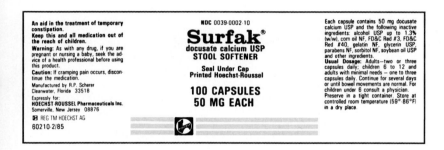

80. Elixir of KC1 15 ml p.o. t.i.d. Elixir of KC1 15 mEq per 11.25 ml is available. How many
mEq will be given? _____ .

81. Phenobarbitol 55 mg p.o. b.i.d. You have phenobarbital gr ¼ per 5. Give _____ .

82. Ilosone 250 mg p.o. q.i.d. Ilosone is supplied in 125 mg capsules. Give _____ .

83. Synthroid 0.05 mg p.o. q. A.M. Synthoid is supplied in 50 mcg tablets. Give _____ .

BOOTS·FLINT

100 Tablets   code 3P1033
(10 Strips -   NDC 0048-1040-13
10 Unit Dose tablets each)

SYNTHROID®

**(Levothyroxine Sodium
Tablets, USP)**

50 mcg (0.05 mg)

Dosage: Adults: Initial - 25 to 100 mcg
(0.025 to 0.1 mg) daily. Usual maintenance dose - 100 to 200 mcg (0.1 to 0.2
mg) daily. Children: Initial - 25 mcg
(0.025 mg) daily. Dosage adjusted by
physician until desired response is obtained. See directions for higher maintenance dosage. SEE ACCOMPANYING
DIRECTIONS.
Keep this and all medications out of the
reach of children.
For hospital use only: Packaging is not
child resistant.
**Caution: Federal (U.S.A.) law
prohibits dispensing without
prescription.**
Manufactured by Boots Puerto Rico, Inc.
Jayuya, Puerto Rico 00664-0795
    For Boots·Flint, Inc.
    Lincolnshire, IL 60015 USA
    a subsidiary of
    The Boots Company (USA) Inc.
            13-1040-02
            11/87

84. Theodur 0.2 Gm p.o. q. 8 h. Theodur is supplied in 100, 200, and 300 mg sustained action tablets. Give _____ tablets of _____ mg. How many mg will be given per day? _____ .

85. Coumadin 15 mg p.o. stat. Coumadin 7.5 mg scored tablets are available. Give _____ .

COUMADIN®
(crystalline warfarin sodium, U.S.P.)
7½ mg
DU PONT PHARMACEUTICALS
Wilmington, Delaware 19898
Lot   X0009A
Exp.   3/88

86. Cimetidine 300 mg p.o. q.i.d. p.c. h.s. How many mg would be given each day? _____ .

87. Restoril 30 mg p.o. h.s. p.r.n. for sleep. You have Restoril 15 mg capsules. How many capsules will you give each h.s.? _____ .

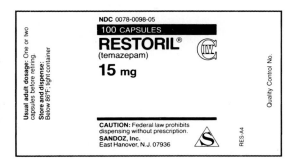

88. Imipramine 50 mg p.o. q. A.M. and h.s. The drug is supplied in 25 mg tablets. Give _____ .

89. Mellaril 40 mg p.o. b.i.d. Mellaril 30 mg per ml is available. Give _____ .

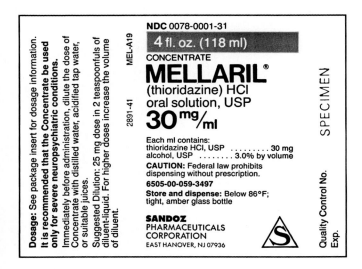

90. Lasix 0.6 ml p.o. b.i.d. with meals. Lasix is available in an oral solution of 10 mg per ml. How many mg will be given? _____ .

91. Cleocin 150 mg p.o. q.6 h. Cleocin is supplied in 75 mg capsules. Give _____ .

92. Crystodigin 0.05 mg p.o. q. A.M. Crystodigin is supplied in 0.1 mg scored tablets. Give _____ .

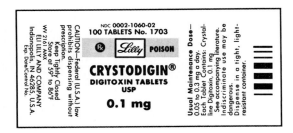

93. Coumadin 10 mg p.o. at 6:00 P.M. today. The drug is supplied in 2.5 mg tablets. Give _____ .

94. Diabinese 0.25 Gm p.o. q. A.M. Diabinese is supplied in 250 mg tablets. Give _____ .

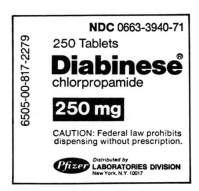

95. Apresoline 25 mg p.o. b.i.d. You have Apresoline tablets gr ⅙. Give _____ .

96. Chloral hydrate elixir 600 mg p.o. h.s. p.r.n. Chloral hydrate 500 mg per 5 ml is available. Give _____ .

97. Prednisone 15 mg p.o. q.d. Prednisone is available in 5 mg tablets. Give _____ .

98. Restoril 0.015 Gm p.o. h.s. for insomnia. You have Restoril 15 mg capsules. Give _____ .

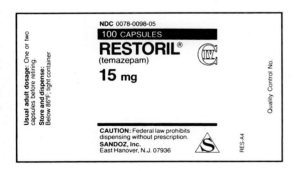

99. KC1 Elixir 40 mEq p.o. q.i.d. c̄ juice. KC1 20 mEq per 15 ml is available. Give _____ .

100. Furosemide 20 mg p.o. q. 8 h. You have Furosemide 40 mg tablets. Give _____ .

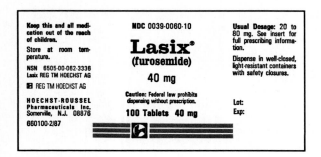

Answers on pp. 357-358.

Name _____

Date _____

ACCEPTABLE SCORE ___18___

YOUR SCORE _____

POSTTEST 1

DIRECTIONS: The medication order is listed at the beginning of each problem. Calculate the oral dosages by the use of a proportion. Show your work. Place your answer in the space provided and label.

1. A.S.A. gr xv p.o. q.i.d. A.S.A. 325 mg tablets are available. Give _____ .

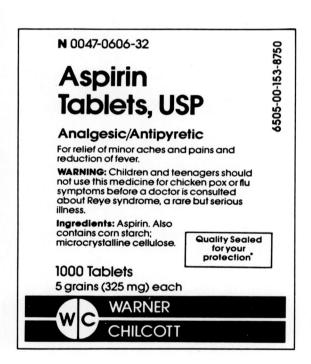

2. Tetracycline 0.5 Gm p.o. q.i.d. The drug is supplied in 500 mg capsules. Give _____ .

3. Ampicillin 1 Gm p.o. q. 6 h. You have 500 mg capsules. Give _____ .

4. Milk of Magnesia 1 Tbsp p.o. h.s. Give _____ ℥.

5. Orinase 500 mg p.o. t.i.d. You have 0.5 Gm tablets available. Give _____ .

6. Atarax 25 mg p.o. q.A.M. You have Atarax 10 mg per 5 ml. Give _____ .

7. Mellaril 30 mg p.o. t.i.d. p.r.n. Mellaril 15 mg tablets are available. Give _____ .

8. Codeine 30 mg p.o. q. 3 h. p.r.n. You have codeine tablets gr ½. Give _____ .

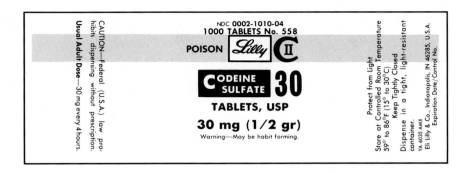

9. Vistaril 50 mg p.o. t.i.d. Vistaril Oral Suspension 25 mg per teaspoon is available. Give
_____ .

10. Naprosyn 0.25 Gm p.o. b.i.d. Naprosyn is supplied in 250 mg scored tablets. How many
Gm will you give each day? _____ .

11. Crystodigin gr ⅟₆₀₀ p.o. q.d. Crystodigin tablets gr ⅟₃₀₀ are available. Give _____ .

12. KC1 20 mEq p.o. b.i.d. KC1 liquid is supplied 30 mEq per 22.5 ml. Give _____ .

13. Gantrisin 2 Gm p.o. t.i.d. You have 500 mg tablets available. Give _____ .

14. Benadryl 100 mg p.o. h.s. p.r.n. Benadryl capsules 50 mg are available. Give _____ .

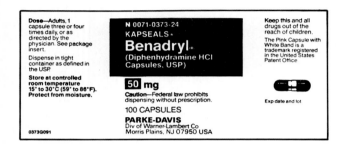

15. Lasix 9 mg p.o. q. 12 h. You have Lasix 10 mg per ml. Give _____ .

16. Keflex 100 mg p.o. q. 6 h. Keflex Oral Suspension 125 mg per 5 ml is available. Give _____ .

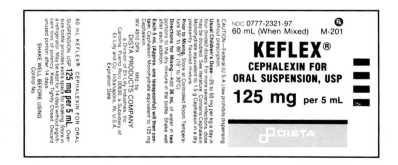

17. Achromycin ℥ ii p.o. q. 6 h. You have a ℥ ii bottle of Achromycin Syrup containing 125 mg per teaspoon. How many mg will be given? _____ .

18. Inderal 80 mg p.o. b.i.d. You have Inderal 40 mg scored tablets. Give _____ .

19. Apresoline 20 mg p.o. t.i.d. You have 10 mg tablets available. Give _____ .

20. Phenobarbital gr iss p.o. t.i.d. You have 60 mg tablets available. How many tablets will you give for each dose? _____ . How many tablets will you need for one day? _____ .

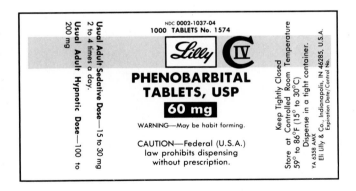

Answers on p. 358.

Name _____

Date _____

ACCEPTABLE SCORE ___18___

YOUR SCORE _____

POSTTEST 2

DIRECTIONS: The medication order is listed at the beginning of each problem Calculate the oral dosages by the use of a proportion. Show your work. Place your answer in the space provided and label.

1. Feldene 20 mg p.o. q.d. Feldene capsules 10 mg are available. Give _____ .

2. Robitussin ʒ ii p.o. q. 4 h. Robitussin is supplied in ʒ iv bottles. How many ʒ ii doses will each bottle provide? _____ .

3. Tylenol Elixir 30 mg p.o. stat. You have Children's Tylenol Elixir 160 mg per 5 ml. Give _____ ℳ.

4. Dicumarol 150 mg p.o. stat. Dicumarol is supplied in 50 mg grooved tablets. Give _____ .

5. KCl 5 mEq p.o. b.i.d. KCl 20 mEq per 30 ml is available. Give _____ .

6. Keflex 250 mg p.o. q.i.d. You have Keflex 0.25 Gm capsules. Give _____ .

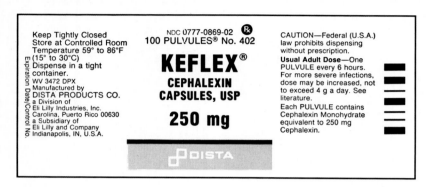

7. Prednisone 7.5 mg p.o. q.i.d. from a supply of 2.5 mg tablets. Give _____ .

8. Lanoxin 0.05 mg p.o. q.d. You have Lanoxin Elixir 0.05 mg per ml. Give _____ .

9. Macrodantin 0.1 Gm p.o. q.i.d. You have Macrodantin 50 mg capsules. Give _____ .

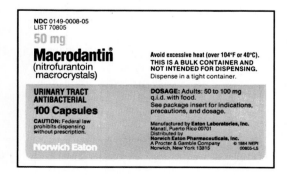

10. Tylenol gr vi p.o. q. 4 h. p.r.n. for pain. Tylenol is supplied in 325 mg tablets. Give
_____ .

11. Dilantin gr ¾ p.o. b.i.d. Dilantin 50 mg Infatabs are available. Give _____ .

12. Pen-Vee K 250 mg p.o. q. 6 h. Pen-Vee K Solution 125 mg per 5 ml is available. Give
_____ .

13. Deltasone 20 mg p.o. q.i.d. Deltasone is supplied in 2.5, 5, and 50 Gm tablets. Give
_____ tablets of _____ mg.

14. Lanoxin 0.25 mg p.o. q.d. You have Lanoxin 0.125 mg tablets. Give _____ .

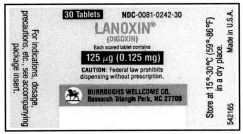

15. Colace Elixir 25 ml p.o. p.r.n. You have Colace Elixir 20 mg per 5 ml. How many mg of Colace will be given? _____ .

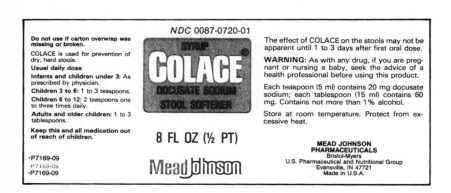

16. A.S.A. 0.6 Gm p.o. q. 3 h. p.r.n. You have A.S.A. gr v tablets. Give _____ .

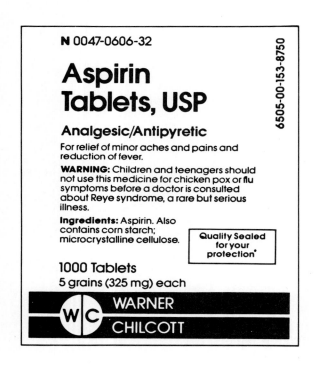

17. Noctec 500 mg p.o. h.s. You have Notec Syrup gr viiss per ℥. Give _____ .

18. Gantrisin tablets 1.5 Gm p.o. q.i.d. Gantrisin 0.5 Gm tablets are supplied. Give _____ .

19. Phenobarbital 30 mg p.o. q. 8 h. You have phenobarbital 15 mg tablets. Give _____ .

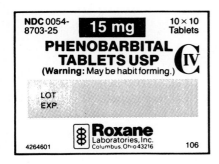

20. Flagyl 750 mg p.o. t.i.d. × 5 days. Flagyl is supplied in 250 mg tablets. Give _____ .

Answers on p. 358.

Name _____

Date _____

ACCEPTABLE SCORE ____18____

YOUR SCORE _____

PRETEST

DIRECTIONS: The medication order is listed at the beginning of each problem. Calculate the parenteral dosages by the use of a proportion. Show your work.

1. Codeine gr ss I.M. q. 4 h. Codeine 0.03 Gm per ml is available. Give _____ .

2. Ampicillin 1 ml I.M. q. 6 h. Ampicillin 2.5 Gm per 10 ml. is available. How many mg will you give? _____ .

3. Scopolamine 0.3 mg I.M. stat. You have Scopolamine gr 1/150 per ml. Give _____ .

4. Dilaudid 3 mg I.M. q. 3 hr. Dilaudid is supplied in 1 ml ampules containing 4 mg. Give _____ .

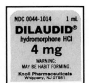

5. Tobramycin 40 mg I.M. q. 8 hr. Tobramycin 60 mg per 1.5 ml is supplied. Give _____ .

6. Morphine gr ⅙ subq. q. 4 h. p.r.n. Morphine 15 mg per ml is available. Give _____ ℳ.

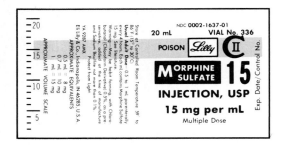

7. Vistaril 100 mg I.M. q. 4 h. p.r.n. Vistaril is supplied in a 10 ml vial containing 50 mg per ml. Give _____ .

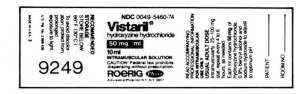

8. Kefzol 500 mg I.M. q. 6 h. Kefzol 225 mg per ml is available. Give _____ .

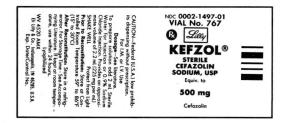

9. Valium 40 mg I.V. stat. Valium 50 mg per 10 ml is supplied. Give _____ .

10. Stadol 0.5 mg I.V. q. 4 h. Stadol 1 mg per ml is available. Give _____ .

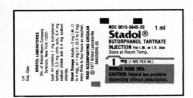

11. Gentamicin 23 mg I.V. q. 8 hr. You have Gentamicin 40 mg per ml available. Prepare _____ .

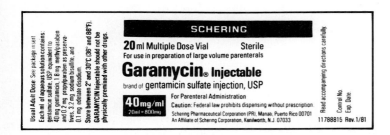

12. Lanoxin 40 mcg I.M. q. 12 h. Lanoxin 0.1 mg per ml is available. Give _____ .

13. Hydrocortisone 8 mg I.V. q. 4 h. The drug is available in a vial containig 100 mg per 2 ml. Prepare _____ ℳ.

14. Atropine gr ¹⁄₁₅₀ I.M. at 9 A.M. You have atropine 0.4 mg per ml available. Give _____ .

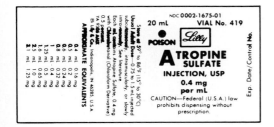

15. Demerol 22 mg I.M. stat. Demerol 25 mg per 0.5 ml is available. Give _____ .

16. Meperidine 0.2 ml I.M. q. 4 h. p.r.n. The drug is supplied in an ampule containing 50 mg per ml. How many mg will you give? _____ .

17. Phenergan 10.5 mg I.M. t.i.d. Phenergan 25 mg per ml is available. Give _____ .

18. Depo-Medrol 50 mg I.M. q. 6 h. The drug is supplied in a vial containing 80 mg per ml. Give _____ .

```
NDC 0009-0306-01          For IM, intrasynovial and soft
1 ml                      tissue injection only.
                          Not for IV use.
Depo-Medrol®              See package insert for
Sterile Aqueous Suspension   complete product
sterile methylprednisolone   information.
acetate suspension, USP   Shake well immediately
                          before using
80 mg per ml              812 312 201
                          The Upjohn Company
                          Kalamazoo, MI 49001, USA
```

19. Synkayvite 10 mg I.M. h.s. Synkayvite is available in a 1 ml ampule containing 5 mg of the drug. Give _____ .

20. D_5W 500 ml plus NaCl 20 mEq at 19 ml per hr. NaCl is supplied in a 40 ml ampule containing 2.5 mEq per ml. How many ml of NaCl will be added to the 500 ml of D_5W? _____ .

Answers on p. 358.

CHAPTER 11

PARENTERAL DOSAGES

Learning objectives

On completion of the materials provided in this chapter, you will be able to perform computations accurately by mastering the following mathematical concepts.

1. Convert the measure within the problem to equivalent measures in one system of measurement
2. Use a proportion to solve problems of parenteral dosages when medication is in liquid or reconstituted powder form.
3. Use a proportion to solve problems of parenteral dosages of medications measured in milliequivalents

Parenteral refers to outside the alimentary canal or the gastrointestinal tract. Medications may be given parenterally when they cannot be taken by mouth or when a rapid action is desired. Parenteral medications are absorbed directly into the bloodstream; therefore the amount of the drug needed can be determined more accurately. This type of administration of medications is necessary for the irrational or unconscious patient or for a patient who has been designated *NPO* (nothing by mouth). Parenterally given drugs also have the advantage of not upsetting the gastrointestinal system.

Parenteral medications are administered by (1) subcutaneous injections—beneath the skin, (2) intramuscular injections—within the muscle; or (3) intravenous injections—within the vein. Intravenous drugs may be diluted and administered by themselves or in conjunction with existing intravenous fluids or added to the IV fluids. At any time that the integrity of the skin, the body's prime defense against microorganisms, is threatened, infection may occur. The nurse must use sterile technique when preparing and administering the parenteral medications.

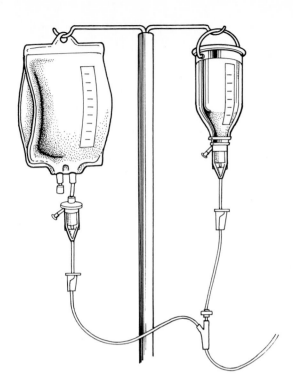

Drugs for parenteral use are supplied as liquids or powders. The medications are packaged in a variety of forms. First, a liquid may be contained in an ampule. An ampule is a single-dose glass container that one must break at the neck to withdraw the drug.

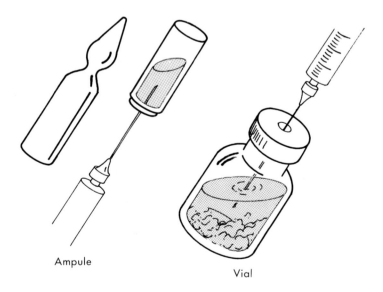

Ampule

Vial

Vials are also used to package parenteral medications in liquid or powder form. A vial is a glass or plastic container that is sealed with a rubber stopper. Since vials usually contain more than one dose of a medication, the amount desired is withdrawn by inserting the needle through the rubber stopper and withdrawing the required amount. If the medication is in powder form, the drug must be reconstituted before withdrawal and administration. The diluent to dissolve the powder is usually sterile water or normal saline. The amount of diluent recommended is normally printed on the vial; however, if it is not, no less than 1 ml is used for a single-dose vial. The powder must be completely dissolved. If one is using a multiple-dose vial, the data and time of mixing should be noted on the vial's label.

Some of the more unstable drugs may be supplied in vials that have a compartment containing the liquid. Pressure applied to the top of the vial releases the stopper between the compartments and allows the drug to be dissolved. These are known as Mix-O-Vials.

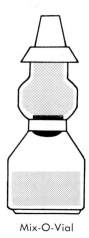

Mix-O-Vial

Prefilled disposable syringes or a plastic syringe (Tubex) with a disposable cartridge with needle unit may be the method by which the drug is supplied. Those units contain a specific amount of medication. If the medication order is less than the amount supplied, discard the unneeded portion before administering the medication to the patient.

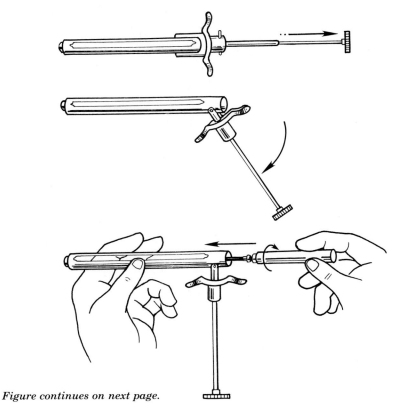

Figure continues on next page.

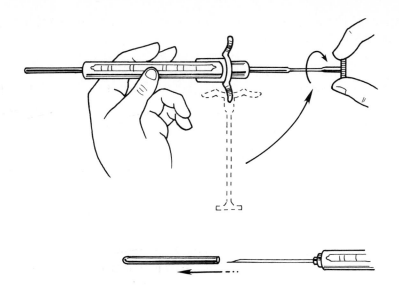

Parenteral drug dosages may also be calculated by the use of a proportion. It remains necessary for the order and the available medication to be in the same system of measurement for one to write a proportion for the actual amount of medication to be administered. Examples of parenteral drug dosage problems follow.

EXAMPLE: Apresoline 30 mg I.M. now Apresoline 20 mg per ml is available. Give _____ .

a. On the left side of the proportion place what you know or have available. In this example there are 20 mg per 1 ml. Therefore, the left side of the proportion would be

$$20 \text{ mg}:1 \text{ ml}::$$

b. The right side of the proportion is determined by the physician's order and the abbreviations placed on the left side of the proportion. Remember, only *two* different abbreviations may be used in a single proportion.

$$20 \text{ mg}:1 \text{ ml}:: \text{_____} \text{ mg}: \text{_____} \text{ ml}$$

The physician ordered 30 mg.

$$20 \text{ mg}:1 \text{ ml}::30 \text{ mg}: \text{_____} \text{ ml}$$

The symbol x is used to represent the unknown number of ml.

$$20 \text{ mg}:1 \text{ ml}::30 \text{ mg}:x \text{ ml}$$

c. Rewrite the proportion without the abbreviations.

$$20:1::30:x$$

d. Solve for x.

$$20:1::30:x$$

$$20x = 30$$

$$x = \frac{30}{20}$$

$$x = 1.5$$

e. Label your answer as determined by the abbreviation placed next to x in the original proportion.

1.5 ml

The patient would receive 1.5 ml of Apresoline containing 30 mg.

EXAMPLE: Demerol 30 mg I.M. q. 4 h. p.r.n. Demerol 25 mg per 0.5 ml is available. Give _____ .

a. On the left side of the proportion place what you know or have available. In this example each 0.5 ml contains 25 mg. So the left side of the proportion would be

25 mg:0.5 ml::

b. The right side of the proportion is determined by the physician's order and the abbreviations on the left side of the proportion. Only *two* different abbreviations may be used in a single proportion. The abbreviations must be in the same position on the right side as they are on the left.

25 mg:0.5 ml:: _____ mg: _____ ml

In this example the physician ordered 30 mg.

25 mg:0.5 ml::30 mg: _____ ml

Since we need to find the number of milliliters to be given, we use the symbol x to represent the unknown.

25 mg:0.5 ml::30 mg:x ml

c. Rewrite the proportion without using the abbreviations.

25:0.5::30:x

d. Solve for x.

$$25x = 0.5 \times 30$$
$$25x = 15$$
$$x = \frac{15}{25}$$
$$x = 0.6$$

e. Label your answer as determined by the abbreviation placed next to x in the original proportion.

0.6 ml would be measured in order to administer 30 mg of Demerol.

If the question asks for the answer to be in minims, another proportion must be written and solved using your new knowledge.

a. 15♏:1 ml::
b. 15♏:1 ml:: _____ ♏ : _____ ml
   15♏:1 ml::x♏:0.6 ml
c. 15:1::x:0.6
d. $x = 9$
e. $x = 9$ ♏

EXAMPLE: Gentamicin 9 mg IV q. 6 h. Gentamicin 20 mg per 2 ml is available. Give
_____ m.

a. 20 mg:2 ml::
b. 20 mg:2 ml:: _____ mg: _____ ml
   20 mg:2 ml::9 mg:x ml
c. 20:2::9:x
d. 20:2::9:x

$$20x = 18$$

$$x = \frac{18}{20}$$

$$x = 0.9$$

$$x = 0.9 \text{ ml.}$$

Since the question asks for the answer to be in minims, another proportion must be written and solved using your new knowledge.

a. 15 m:1 ml::
b. 15 m:1 ml:: _____ m: _____ ml
   15 m:1 ml::xm:0.9 ml
c. 15:1::x:0.9
d. $x = 13.5$
e. $x = 13.5$ m

Complete the following work sheet, which provides for extensive practice in the calculation of parenteral drug dosage problems. Check your answers. If you have difficulties, go back and review the necessary material. When you feel ready to evaluate your learning, take the first posttest. Check your answers. An acceptable score as indicated on the posttest signifies that you have successfully completed this chapter. An unacceptable score signifies a need for further study before taking the second posttest.

WORK SHEET

The medication order is listed at the beginning of each problem. Calculate the parenteral dosages by the use of a proportion. Show your work.

1. Gentamicin 30 mg I.M. q. 8 h. Gentamicin 10 mg per ml is available. Give _____ .

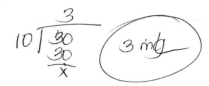

2. Lanoxin 110 mcg I.V. q. 12 h. Lanoxin 0.5 mg per 2 ml is available. Prepare _____ .

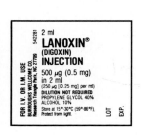
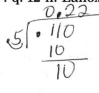
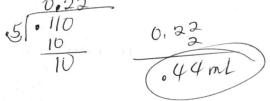

3. Atropine gr ½₀₀ I.M. at 6:15 A.M. Atropine 0.4 mg per ml is available. Give _____ .

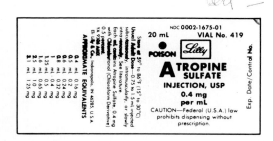
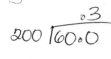
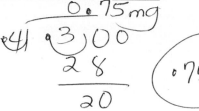

4. Compazine 10 mg I.M. q. 6 h. Compazine is supplied in a 10 ml vial containing 5 mg per ml. Give _____ .

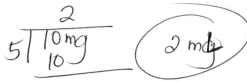

5. Meperidine 45 mg I.M. q. 4 h. Meperidine is supplied in an ampule containing 25 mg per 0.5 ml. Give _____ .

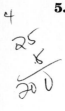

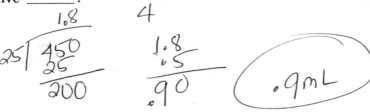

6. Piperacillin 3 Gm I.V. q. 8 h. You have piperacillin 1 Gm per 2.5 ml available. Give _____ .

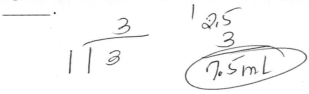

7. Morphine 5 mg subq. q. 4 h. You have morphine gr ⅙ per ml available. Give _____ .

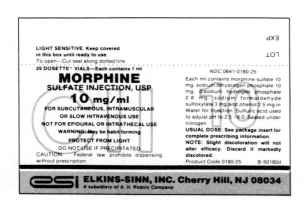

LIGHT SENSITIVE: Keep covered
in this box until ready to use.
To open—Cut seal along dotted line

25 DOSETTE · VIALS—Each contains 1 ml

MORPHINE
SULFATE INJECTION, USP
10 mg/ml
FOR SUBCUTANEOUS, INTRAMUSCULAR
OR SLOW INTRAVENOUS USE
NOT FOR EPIDURAL OR INTRATHECAL USE
WARNING: May be habit forming
PROTECT FROM LIGHT
DO NOT USE IF PRECIPITATED
CAUTION   Federal law prohibits dispensing
without prescription

EXP
LOT

NDC 0641-0180-25

Each ml contains morphine sulfate 10
mg, sodium dihydrogen phosphate 10
mg, disodium hydrogen phosphate
2 8 mg, sodium formaldehyde
sulfoxylate 3 mg and phenol 2 5 mg in
Water for Injection Sulfuric acid used
to adjust pH to 2 5 - 6 0. Sealed under
nitrogen
USUAL DOSE: See package insert for
complete prescribing information.
NOTE: Slight discoloration will not
alter efficacy. Discard if markedly
discolored.
Product Code 0180-25   B-50180d

ELKINS-SINN, INC. Cherry Hill, NJ 08034
A subsidiary of A. H. Robins Company

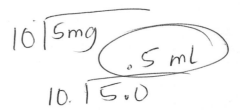

8. Vancomycin 1 Gm I.V. SS q. 12 h. After reconstitution of the medication, you have Vancomycin 500 mg per 6 ml. Give _____ .

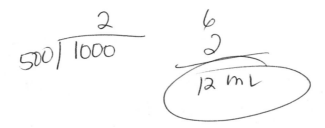

9. Lasix 30 mg I.M. stat. Lasix is supplied in a 2 ml ampule containing 10 mg per ml. Give _____ .

$$10\overline{)30} \quad \frac{3}{}$$

$$\boxed{3\,mL}$$

10. Morphine gr ¼₄ subq. q. 4 h. You have morphine gr ⅛ per 30 ℳ available. Give _____ .

$$24\overline{)1000}\;\;\frac{2}{} \\ 48 \\ \overline{120}$$

11. D₅W 1000 ml plus NaHCO₃ 25.8 mEq at 12 ml per h. NaHCO₃ is supplied in a 50 ml ampule containing 44.6 mEq. How many ml of NaHCO₃ will be added to the 1000 ml of D₅W? _____ .

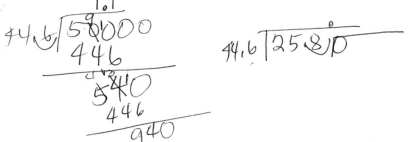

$$44.6\overline{)50000}\;\;1.1 \\ 446 \\ 540 \\ 446 \\ \overline{940}$$

$$44.6\overline{)2580}$$

12. Aminophylline 100 mg I.V. q. 6 h. You have aminophylline 500 mg per 20 ml available. Give _____ .

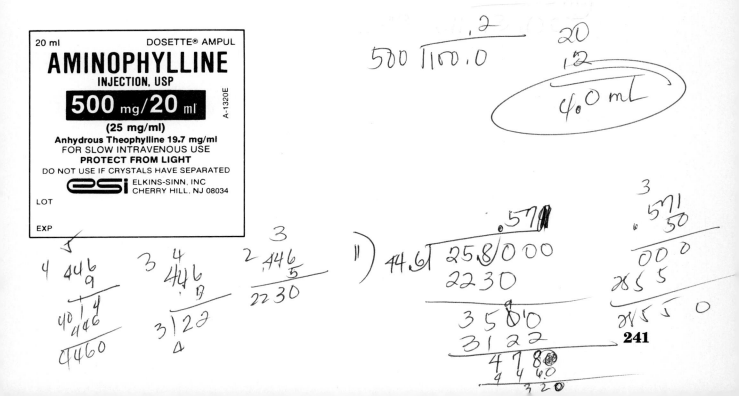

$$20\,ml \quad \text{DOSETTE® AMPUL}$$

AMINOPHYLLINE
INJECTION, USP

500 mg/20 ml A-1320E

(25 mg/ml)
Anhydrous Theophylline 19.7 mg/ml
FOR SLOW INTRAVENOUS USE
PROTECT FROM LIGHT
DO NOT USE IF CRYSTALS HAVE SEPARATED
eSi ELKINS-SINN, INC
CHERRY HILL, NJ 08034

LOT

EXP

$$500\overline{)1100.0}\;\;.2 \qquad \frac{20}{12}$$

$$\boxed{4.0\,mL}$$

$$4\overline{)446}\;\frac{}{9} \\ 40 \\ 44\,4 \\ 446 \\ \overline{4460}$$

$$3\overline{)446}\;\frac{4}{} \\ 44\,6 \\ 3\overline{)22} \\ A$$

$$\frac{3}{2.446}\times 5 \\ \overline{2230}$$

$$11)\;44.6\overline{)25.80000}\;.57 \\ 2230 \\ 3580 \\ 3122 \\ 478\,60 \\ \overline{320}$$

$$\frac{3}{.571}\,50 \\ \overline{000} \\ 2855 \\ 2855\;0$$

13. Dilaudid gr ¹⁄₁₅ subq q. 3 h. You have Dilaudid 2 mg per ml available. Give _____ ℳ.

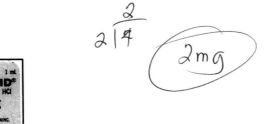

$$2\overline{)4} \quad \frac{2}{}$$

(2 mg)

14. Gantrisin gr xv I.V. stat. You have a 5 ml ampule containing 2 Gm. Prepare _____ .

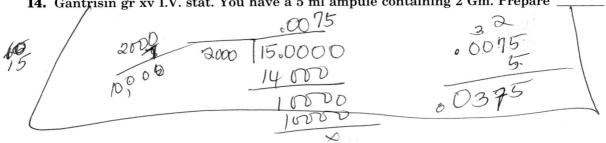

15. Solu-Cortef 0.05 Gm I.M. q. 6 h. You have Solu-Cortef 250 mg per 2 ml. Give _____ .

16. Phenobarbital 0.3 Gm I.M. t.i.d. Phenobarbital 120 mg per ml is available. Give _____ .

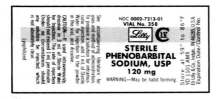

17. Tagamet 300 mg I.V. SS q. 6 h. The drug is supplied in a single dose vial with 300 mg per 2 ml. Give _____ .

18. Hydrocortisone 8 mg I.M. q.d. You have hydrocortisone 100 mg per 2 ml. Give _____ ℳ.

19. Stadol 0.5 mg I.M. q. 4 h. You have Stadol 2 mg per ml. Give _____ .

20. Ativan 0.5 mg I.M. stat. You have Ativan 2 mg per ml. Give _____ .

21. Apresoline 10 mg I.M. q. 6 h. The drug is supplied in 1 ml ampules containing 20 mg. Give _____ .

22. D₅W 1000 ml plus KCl 30 mEq at 60 ml per h. KCl is supplied in a 10 ml vial containing 20 mEq. How many ml of KCl will be added to the 1000 ml of D₅W? _____ .

23. Valium 10 mg I.M. q. 6 h. You have Valium 5 mg per ml. Give _____ .

24. Codeine gr ¼ I.M. q. 3 h. p.r.n. You have codeine 30 mg per ml. Give _____ .

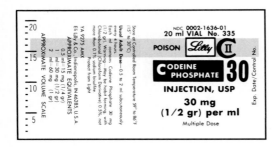

25. AquaMephyton 0.01 Gm I.M. q. A.M. The drug is supplied in 1 ml ampules containing 10 mg per ml. Give _____ .

26. Carbenicillin 6 Gm I.V. SS q. 6 h. You have carbenicillin 2 Gm per 6 ml. Give _____ .

27. Morphine 12 mg I.M. q. 4 h. p.r.n. You have morphine 15 mg per ml. Give _____ .

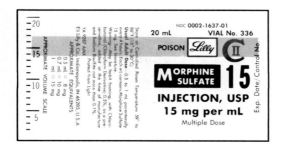

28. Benadryl 100 mg I.M. q.i.d. The drug is supplied in ampules containing 50 mg per ml. Give _____ .

29. Digoxin 100 mcg I.M. q.d. The drug is supplied 0.5 mg per 2 ml. Give _____ .

30. Kefzol 500 mg I.V. SS q. 6 h. × 4 days. Kefzol 225 mg per ml is available. Give _____ .

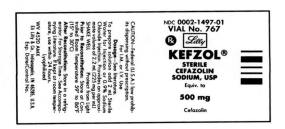

31. Phenobarbital gr v I.M. q. 3 h. You have 120 mg per ml. Give _____ .

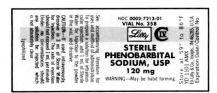

32. Solu-Cortef 100 mg I.M. q. 8 h. Solu-Cortef 250 mg per 2 ml is available. Give _____ .

33. D_5W 250 ml plus NaCl 7.5 mEq at 2 ml per h. NaCl is supplied in a 40 ml vial containing 2.5 mEq per ml. How many ml of NaCl will be added to the 250 ml of D_5W? _____ .

34. Vistaril 3 ml I.M. t.i.d. You have Vistaril 50 mg per ml available. How many mg will you give? _____ .

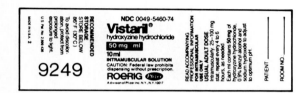

35. Atropine gr $\frac{1}{100}$ I.M. stat. You have atropine gr $\frac{1}{150}$ per ml available. Give _____ .

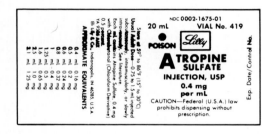

36. Seconal 50 mg I.M. h.s. p.r.n. You have a 5 ml vial containing 250 mg of the drug. Give _____ .

37. Demerol 75 mg I.M. q. 4 h. p.r.n. Demerol is supplied in a 2 ml ampule containing 100 mg of the drug. Give _____ .

38. Aminophylline 75 mg I.V. q. 6 h. You have aminophylline 25 mg per ml. Prepare _____ .

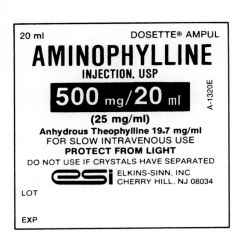

39. Librium 75 mg I.M. stat. Librium 100 mg per 2 ml is available. Give _____ .

40. Valium 15 mg I.V. stat. Valium is supplied in a 10 ml vial containing 5 mg per ml. Prepare _____ .

41. Hydrocortisone 25 mg I.M. q.d. The drug is available 100 mg per 2 ml. Give _____ .

42. Kantrex 400 mg I.M. q. 12 h. You have Kantrex 500 mg per 2 ml. available. Give
_____ .

43. Ascorbic acid 0.25 Gm I.M. q.d. You have ascorbic acid 500 mg per ml. Give _____ .

44. D_5W 250 ml plus $CaCl_2$ 5 mEq at 2 ml per h. $CaCl_2$ is supplied in a 10 ml ampule containing 13.6 mEq. How many ml of $CaCl_2$ will be added to the 250 ml of D_5W? _____ .

45. Phenobarbital 70 mg subq. q. 8 h. The drug is supplied in a 1 ml ampule containing 65 mg. Give _____ .

46. Vibramycin 200 mg I.V. q.d. You have Vibramycin 10 mg per ml after reconstitution. Give _____ .

47. Dilaudid gr 1/30 I.M. q. 4 h. p.r.n. Dilaudid 4 mg per ml is available. Give _____ .

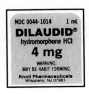

48. Digoxin 0.2 mg I.M. q.d. The drug is available in a 2 ml ampule containing 0.5 mg. Give _____ .

49. Morphine gr 1/6 subq. q. 3 h. Morphine is available in an ampule containing gr 1/4 per ml. Give _____ ℳ.

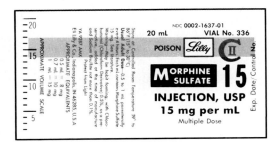

50. Haldol 3 mg I.M. q.i.d. The drug is supplied in a 1 ml ampule containing 5 mg. Give _____ ℳ.

51. Demerol 0.6 ml I.M. q 3 h. p.r.n. Demerol is supplied in a 30 ml vial containing 50 mg per ml. How many mg will you give? _____ .

52. Atropine 0.9 mg I.M. at 6:15 A.M. You have atropine gr ⅟₂₀₀ per ml available. Give _____ .

53. Codeine gr ss subq. q. 4 h. Codeine 30 mg per ml is available. Give _____ .

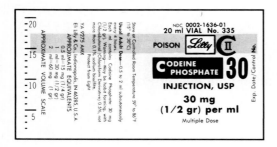

54. Phenobarbital gr ¼ subq. q. 3 h. Phenobarbital is supplied in 1 ml ampules containing 65 mg. Give _____ ♏︎.

55. D_5W 500 ml plus 6 mEq of $NaHCO_3$ at 42 ml per h. $NaHCO_3$ is available in a 10 ml ampule containing 0.89 mEq per ml. How many ml of $NaHCO_3$ will be added to the 500 ml of D_5W? _____ .

56. Garamycin 20 mg I.M. q. 8 h. Garamycin is supplied in a 2 ml vial containing 40 mg per ml. Give _____ .

SCHERING

Usual Adult Dose See package insert

Each ml of aqueous solution contains: gentamicin sulfate, USP equivalent to 40 mg gentamicin, 1.8 mg methylparaben and 0.2 mg propylparaben as preservatives, 3.2 mg sodium bisulfite, and 0.1 mg edetate disodium

Store between 2° and 30°C (36° and 86°F). GARAMYCIN Injectable should not be physically premixed with other drugs.

20 ml Multiple Dose Vial   Sterile
For use in preparation of large volume parenterals

Garamycin® Injectable
brand of gentamicin sulfate injection, USP

40 mg/ml
20ml = 800mg

For Parenteral Administration
Caution: Federal law prohibits dispensing without prescription.
Schering Pharmaceutical Corporation (PR), Manati, Puerto Rico 00701
An Affiliate of Schering Corporation, Kenilworth, N.J. 07033

Read accompanying directions carefully

Control No
Exp. Date

11788815 Rev.1/81

57. Thorazine 0.2 ml I.M. q. 4 h. You have Thorazine 25 mg per ml. How many mg will you give? _____ .

58. Ampicillin 500 mg I.V. SS q. 12 h. You have ampicillin 100 mg per ml. Give _____ .

59. Demerol 50 mg I.M. q. 4 h. p.r.n. Demerol is supplied in a vial containing 100 mg per ml. Give _____ .

60. Ativan 0.5 mg I.M. stat. The drug is supplied in a 1 ml vial containing 2 mg per ml. Give _____ .

61. Aminophylline 0.2 Gm I.V. t.i.d. Aminophylline is supplied in a 10 ml ampule containing 0.25 Gm per 10 ml. Give _____ .

62. Codeine 15 mg I.M. q. 4 h. Codeine is available in an ampule containing gr ss per ml. Give _____ .

63. Dilantin 100 mg I.V. q. 8 h. You have available Dilantin 50 mg per ml. Give _____ .

64. Digoxin 0.25 mg I.V. q.d. Digoxin is supplied in a 2 ml ampule containing 0.5 mg. Give _____ .

65. Demerol 35 mg I.M. q. 3 h. for severe pain. The drug is supplied in an ampule containing 25 mg per 0.5 ml. Give _____ .

66. $D_{7,5}W$ 250 ml plus calcium gluconate 5 mEq at 2 ml per h. Calcium gluconate is supplied in a 10 ml ampule containing 4.8 mEq. How many ml of calcium gluconate will be added to the 250 ml of $D_{7,5}W$? _____ .

67. Cleocin 50 mg I.V. q. 8 h. Cleocin is available in a 2 ml ampule containing 300 mg. Give _____ .

68. Atropine 0.2 mg I.M. at 7:30 A.M. Atropine is supplied in a 1 ml ampule containing 1 mg. Give _____ .

69. Tobramycin 55 mg I.V. q. 8 h. You have Tobramycin 40 mg per ml available. Give _____ .

70. Phenobarbital 22 mg I.M. as an anticonvulsant. Phenobarbital is supplied in 1 ml ampules contaning 65 mg. Give _____ .

71. Morphine 10 mg subq. stat. Morphine is supplied in a 20 ml vial containing ¼ gr per ml. Give _____ ℳ.

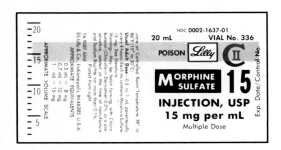

72. Vitamin B$_{12}$ 1 mg I.M. q. Monday. Vitamin B$_{12}$ is available in a 10 ml vial containing 1000 mcg per ml. Give _____ .

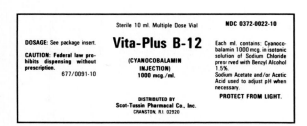

73. Morphine gr ¹⁄₃₀ I.M. q. 3 h. Morphine is available in an ampule containing gr ⅛ per ml. Give _____ ℳ.

74. Phenergan 6.5 mg I.M. at 9:30 A.M. Phenergan is supplied in an ampule containing 25 mg per ml. Give _____ .

75. Robinul 0.28 mg I.M. at 6:00 A.M. You have a multiple-dose vial with 0.2 mg per ml. Give _____ .

```
┌─────────────────────────────────────────────────────────────┐
│ 5 mL Multiple Dose Vial  NDC 0031-7890-93   CAUTION: Federal law prohibits dispens- │
│ Robinul® Injectable       ing without prescription.          │
│ (Glycopyrrolate Injection, USP)   For I.M. or I.V. administration.   │
│        0.2 mg/mL          For dosage and other directions for use,  │
│ Water for Injection, USP q.s./Benzyl   consult accompanying product literature.  │
│ Alcohol, NF (preservative) 0.9%.   Store at Controlled Room Temperature.  │
│ [ NOT FOR USE IN NEWBORNS ]   Between 15°C and 30°C (59°F and 86°F).  │
│ pH adjusted, when necessary, with hydro-   MANUFACTURED FOR PHARMACEUTICAL DIVISION  │
│ chloric acid and/or sodium hydroxide.   A.H. ROBINS COMPANY, RICHMOND, VA. 23220  │
│                           by ELKINS-SINN, INC., CHERRY HILL, N.J. 08003  │
│                           a subsidiary of A.H. Robins      10.87  │
└─────────────────────────────────────────────────────────────┘
```

76. Demerol 10 mg I.M q. 6 h. Demerol is available in an ampule containing 25 mg per ml. Give _____ .

77. D_5W 1000 ml plus NaCl 15 mEq at 30 ml per h. NaCl is supplied in a 40 ml vial containing 100 mEq. How many ml of NaCl will be added to the 1000 ml of D_5W? _____ .

78. Kefzol 250 mg I.V. q. 6 h. for 12 doses. The drug is available in a vial containing 125 mg per ml. Give _____ .

79. Cleocin 300 mg I.V. q. 6 h. Cleocin is available in a 4 ml ampule containing 600 mg. Give _____ .

80. Lidocaine 75 mg I.V. stat. Lidocaine is available is a 5 ml vial containing 100 mg per 5 ml. Give _____ ℳ.

81. Sodium phenobarbital 20 mg I.M. b.i.d. The drug is supplied in an ampule containing gr ii per ml. Give _____ .

82. Solu-Medrol 100 mg I.V. stat. The drug is supplied in a Mix-O-Vial containing 125 mg per 2 ml. Give _____ .

83. Demerol 25 mg I.M. on call to O.R. Demerol is available in an ampule containing 50 mg per ml. Give _____ .

84. Scopolamine gr 1/150 at 7 A.M. Scopolamine 0.4 mg per ml is available. Give _____ ℳ.

85. Phenergan 0.2 ml I.M. stat. Phenergan is supplied in an ampule containing 25 mg per ml. Give _____ mg.

86. Dilaudid gr ¹⁄₆₀ q. 4 h. p.r.n. You have an ampule containing Diluadid 10 mg per ml. Give

_____ .

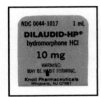

87. Vistaril 50 mg I.M. q. 4 h. p.r.n. for severe agitation. Vistaril is supplied in a 2 ml vial containing 100 mg. Give _____ .

88. D_5W 500 ml plus KCl 10.8 mEq at 42 ml per h. KCl is supplied in a 20 ml vial containing 2 mEq per ml. How many ml of KCl will be added to the 500 ml of D_5W? _____ .

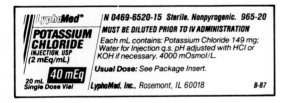

89. Atropine gr ¹⁄₁₂₀ I.M. stat. Atropine is available in an ampule containing gr ¹⁄₁₅₀ per ml. Give _____ ℳ.

90. Thorazine 15 mg I.M. q. 6 hr. p.r.n. Thorazine is supplied in a 10 ml vial containing 25 mg per ml. Give _____ .

91. Vancocin 500 mg I.V. SS q. 12 h. Vancocin 250 mg per 5 ml is available after reconstitution. Give _____ .

NDC 0002-1444-01
VIAL No. 657
℞ Lilly
VANCOCIN®HCl
sterile vancomycin
hydrochloride, usp
INTRAVENOUS
Equiv. to
500 mg
Vancomycin

FOR INTRAVENOUS USE
IMPORTANT—Read literature
for precautions and directions
before use.
Usual Adult Dose—2 g daily.
Dilute with 10 ml of Sterile
Water for Injection.
After Dilution—Refrigerate.
Prior to Reconstitution Store at
59° to 86°F.
MUST BE FURTHER DILUTED
BEFORE USE—SEE LITERATURE
Lyophilized
YD 2651 AMX Mfd. by
Eli Lilly Industries, Inc.
Carolina, Puerto Rico 00630, a subsidiary of
Eli Lilly & Co., Indianapolis, IN, U.S.A.

Exp. Date/Control No.

92. Tobramycin 90 mg I.V. P.B. q. 8 h. You have Tobramycin 80 mg per 2 ml. Give _____ .

93. Valium 2 mg I.M. q. 6 h. Valium is available in a vial containing 5 mg per ml. Give _____ .

94. Flagyl 500 mg I.V. q. 6 h. After reconstitution you have Flagyl 100 mg per ml. Give _____ .

95. Streptomycin 0.64 Gm I.M. q.d. After reconstitution you have Streptomycin 400 mg per ml. Give _____ .

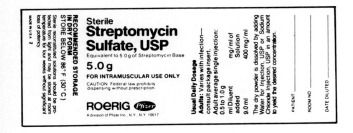

96. Nafcillin 500 mg I.M. q. 6 h. You have nafcillin 250 mg per ml. Give _____ .

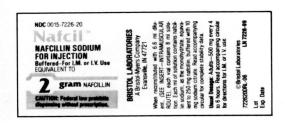

97. Isuprel 0.2 mg stat. I.M. The drug is available in 5 ml ampules containing 1 mg of Isuprel. Give _____ .

98. Imferon 100 mg I.M. q.o.d. The drug is supplied in ampules containing 25 mg per 0.5 ml. Give _____ .

99. Solganal 10 mg I.M. Solganal is supplied 50 mg per ml. Give _____ .

100. Aramine 4 mg I.M. stat. Aramine is available in a vial containing 10 mg per ml. Give _____ .

Answers on pp. 358-359.

Name _____

Date _____

ACCEPTABLE SCORE ___**18**___

YOUR SCORE _____

POSTTEST 1

DIRECTIONS: The medication order is listed at the beginning of each problem. Calculate the parenteral dosages by the use of a proportion. Show your work.

1. Vistaril 50 mg I.M. t.i.d. q. 4-6 h. p.r.n. Vistaril 25 mg per ml is available. Give _____ .

2. Phenergan 5.5 mg I.M. q.i.d. Phenergan 25 mg per ml is available. Give _____ ℳ.

3. Codeine 30 mg I.M. q. 2 h. p.r.n. Codeine is supplied in a 1 ml ampule containing gr ¼ Give _____ .

4. Keflin 500 mg I.M. q. 6 h. Keflin 1 Gm per 10 ml is available. Give _____ .

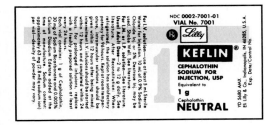

5. Hydrocortisone 50 mg I.M. b.i.d. You have hydrocortisone 100 mg per 2 ml available. Give _____ .

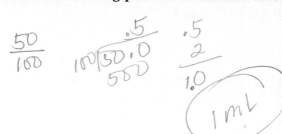

$$\frac{50}{100}$$

$$100\overline{)\begin{array}{c} .5 \\ 50.0 \\ 500 \end{array}}$$

$$\begin{array}{c} .5 \\ 2 \\ \hline 1.0 \end{array}$$

$\boxed{1\,ml}$

6. Dilaudid 0.5 mg I.M. q. 4 h. p.r.n. Dilaudid is supplied in a 1 ml ampule containing 2 mg. Give _____ .

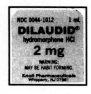

7. Phenobarbital gr iv I.M. b.i.d. Phenobarbital is supplied in a 1 ml ampule containing 120 mg per ml. Give _____ .

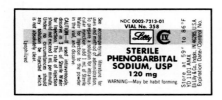

8. Scopolamine gr 1/300 I.M. at 6 A.M. The drug is available in a 1 ml ampule containing 0.4 mg. Give _____ .

9. Thorazine 100 mg I.M. stat. Thorazine is supplied in a 10 ml vial containing 25 mg per ml. Give _____ .

10. Valium 2 mg I.M. q. 6 h. p.r.n. You have a 10 ml vial of the drug containing 5 mg per ml. Give _____ .

11. Atropine 0.7 mg I.M. stat. You have atropine gr $\frac{1}{120}$ per ml. Give _____ .

12. Benadryl 25 mg I.M. p.r.n. You have Benadryl 50 mg per ml available. Give _____ .

13. Demerol 42 mg I.M. q. 4 h. p.r.n. You have an ampule containing 25 mg per 0.5 ml. Give _____ .

14. Ampicillin 500 mg I.M. q. 4 h. You have ampicillin 2.5 Gm per 10 ml available. Give _____ .

15. Librium 0.5 ml I.M. q.i.d. The drug is available in a 5 ml ampule containing 100 mg. How many mg will you give? _____ .

16. Morphine 6 mg I.M. q. 3 h. p.r.n. The drug is supplied in a 1 ml ampule containing gr ⅙. Give _____ .

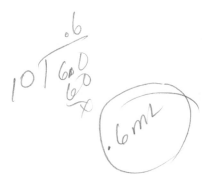

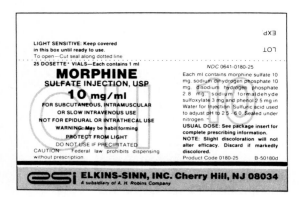

17. Achromycin 300 mg I.V. q. 12 h. Achromycin is supplied in a vial containing 500 mg per 10 ml. Give _____ .

18. Furosemide 10 mg I.M. q. 6 h. Furosemide 20 mg per 2 ml is available. Give _____ .

19. Lanoxin 20 mcg I.M. q. 12 h. You have Lanoxin 0.1 mg per 1 ml. Give _____ ℳ.

20. D$_5$W 500 ml plus KCl 5 mEq at 40 ml per h. KCl is supplied in a 10 ml ampule containing 20 mEq per ml. How many ml of KCl will be added to the 500 ml of D$_5$W? _____ .

$$\frac{5}{20}$$

$$\begin{array}{r} .25 \\ 20\overline{)5.00} \\ 4\ 0 \\ \hline 100 \end{array}$$

.25 mL

Answers on p. 359.

Name _____

Date _____

ACCEPTABLE SCORE ___18___

YOUR SCORE _____

POSTTEST 2

DIRECTIONS: The medication order is listed at the beginning of each problem. Calculate the parenteral dosages by the use of proportions. Show your work.

1. Dilaudid 2 mg I.M. q. 3 h. p.r.n. Dilaudid is supplied in 1 ml ampules containing 4 mg. Give _____ .

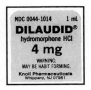

2. Ativan 1 mg I.M. q. 6 h. Ativan 2 mg per ml is available. Give _____ .

3. Erythromycin 0.4 Gm I.V. today. The drug is supplied in vials containing 500 mg per 10 ml. Prepare _____ .

4. Seconal 75 mg I.M. h.s. p.r.n. You have Seconal 250 mg per 5 ml available. Give _____ .

5. Codeine 60 mg I.M. q. 3 h. Codeine gr. ½ per ml is available. Give _____ .

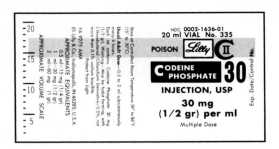

6. Demerol 15 mg I.M. q. 4 h. p.r.n. Demerol is available in an ampule containing 25 mg per 0.5 ml. Give _____ .

7. Atropine gr ½₀₀ I.M. at 6 A.M. You have atropine 0.4 mg per ml. Give _____ .

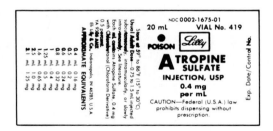

8. Benadryl 25 mg IV. P.B. now. Benadryl 10 mg per ml is available. Give _____ .

9. Tobramycin sulfate 55 mg I.V. q. 8 h. Tobramycin 40 mg per ml is available. Give _____ .

10. Thorazine 30 mg I.M. p.r.n. Thorazine is supplied in 10 ml vial containing 25 mg per ml. Give _____ .

11. Ampicillin 200 mg I.V. q. 6 h. Ampicillin 100 mg per ml is available. Give _____ .

12. Scopolamine gr ¹⁄₁₅₀ I.M. at 7 A.M. Scopolamine gr ¹⁄₂₀₀ per ml is available. Give _____ ℳ.

13. Pipercillin 2 Gm I.V. q. 8 h. Pipercillin 1 Gm per 2.5 ml is available. Give _____ .

14. Gentamicin 26 mg I.V. q. 8 h. Gentamicin 40 mg per ml is available. Prepare _____ ℳ.

Usual Adult Dose See package insert
Each ml of aqueous solution contains:
gentamicin sulfate, USP equivalent to
40 mg gentamicin, 1.8 mg methylparaben
and 0.2 mg propylparaben as preservatives, 3.2 mg sodium bisulfite, and
0.1 mg edetate disodium.

Store between 2° and 30°C (36° and 86°F).
GARAMYCIN Injectable should not be
physically premixed with other drugs.

SCHERING

20 ml Multiple Dose Vial   Sterile
For use in preparation of large volume parenterals

Garamycin® Injectable
brand of **gentamicin sulfate injection, USP**

40 mg/ml
20ml = 800mg

For Parenteral Administration
Caution: Federal law prohibits dispensing without prescription
Schering Pharmaceutical Corporation (PR), Manati, Puerto Rico 00701
An Affiliate of Schering Corporation, Kenilworth, N.J. 07033

11788815 Rev.1/81

Read accompanying directions carefully.

Control No
Exp Date

15. Meperidine 6 ♏ I.M. q. 3 h. p.r.n. The drug is available in an ampule containing 50 mg per ml. How many mg of the drug will you give? _____ .

16. Lanoxin 80 mcg I.M. b.i.d. Lanoxin 0.5 mg per 2 ml is available. Give _____ ♏.

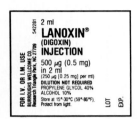

17. Morphine 4 mg subq. q. 4 h. p.r.n. Morphine is supplied in 1 ml ampule containing gr ⅛. Give _____ ♏.

18. Dilantin 100 mg I.V. q. 8 h. Dilantin 50 mg per 2 ml is available. Give _____ .

19. Phenobarbital 0.2 Gm I.M. q. 4 h. Phenobarbital is supplied in a 1 ml ampule containing 120 mg. Give _____ .

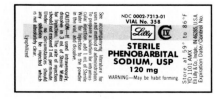

20. D_5W 500 ml plus $CaCl_2$ 10 mEq at 10 ml per h. $CaCl_2$ is supplied in a 10 ml ampule containing 13.6 mEq. How many ml of $CaCl_2$ will be added to the 500 ml of D_5W? _____ .

Answers on p. 359.

PRETEST

DIRECTIONS: The medication order is listed at the beginning of each problem. Calculate the dosages measured in units by the use of a proportion. Show your work.

1. Heparin 5000 U subq. q. 12 h. Heparin 10,000 U per ml is available. Give _____ .

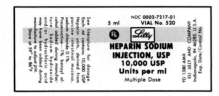

2. Lente insulin 16 U subq. q. A.M. You have lente insulin U-100 and a U-100 syringe. Draw a vertical line through the syringe to indicate the dosage.

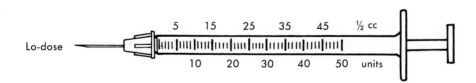

Lo-dose

3. Penicillin V 300,000 U p.o. q.i.d. The drug is supplied in oral solution 200,000 U per 5 ml. Give _____ .

4. NPH insulin 24 U subq. q. A.M. NPH insulin U-100 and a tuberculin syringe are supplied. Give _____ ml.

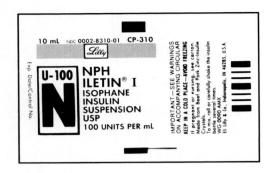

5. Heparin 0.5 ml when I.V. is not infusing. Heparin 10,000 U per ml is available. Give _____ U.

6. Penicillin G 200,000 U I.M. q. 6 h. You have penicillin G 250,000 U per ml. Give _____ .

7. NPH insulin 20 U, regular insulin 5 U subq. q. A.M. NPH insulin U-100, regular insulin U-100, and a U-100 syringe are supplied. Draw a vertical line through the syringe to indicate the amount of NPH insulin to be given, and a second line to indicate the total dosage.

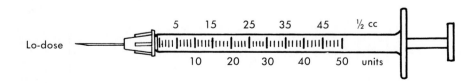

8. Lente insulin 38 U subq. q. A.M. Lente insulin U-100, and a 3 ml syringe are supplied. Give

_____ ℥.

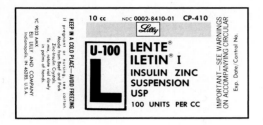

Answers on p. 359

CHAPTER 12

DOSAGES MEASURED IN UNITS

Learning objectives

On completion of the materials provided in this chapter, you will be able to perform computations accurately by mastering the following mathematical concepts:

1. Use a proportion to solve problems involving drugs measured in unit dosages
2. Convert unit dosages of insulin to milliliters or minims
3. Draw a line through an illustration of an insulin syringe to indicate the dosage of units desired

A unit (U) is the amount of a drug needed to produce a given result. Various drugs are measured in units; the examples used in this chapter are among the more common drugs used in hospitals and health care centers on a daily basis.

Drugs used in this chapter include the following:

penicillin antibiotic (reduces organisms within the body that cause infection)

heparin anticoagulant (inhibits clotting of the blood)

insulin hormone secreted by the pancreas, which lowers blood sugar

Penicillin can be administered orally or parenterally, but heparin and insulin must be given subcutaneously.

Before administering penicillin the nurse must confer with the patient regarding previous allergies to the drug. After administration of the drug, the nurse must still observe the patient for signs of an allergic reaction.

Since heparin prolongs the time blood takes to clot, the dosage must be accurate. A larger dose may cause hemorrhage, and an insufficient dose may not have the desired reaction. After the administration of the drug, the nurse should observe the patient for signs of hemorrhage.

Insulin is used in the treatment of diabetes mellitus. Accuracy is important in the preparation of insulin. A higher dose than needed may cause insulin shock; an insufficient amount of insulin could result in diabetic coma. Both conditions are extremely serious, and the nurse must be able to recognize the symptoms of each condition so that immediate treatment can be given to stabilize the patient.

Both insulin and heparin dosages should be observed for accuracy by another nurse before the drug is administered to the patient.

A U-100 insulin syringe and U-100 insulin are necessary to ensure an accurate insulin dosage. U-100 insulin means that 100 U of insulin are contained in 1 ml of liquid. U-100 insulin is a universal insulin preparation that all persons requiring insulin can use. Another type of U-100 syringe is the U-100 low-dose syringe, which measures 50 U; however, for accuracy, no more than 40 U should be measured in the U-100 low-dose syringe. The U-100 syringe is the most accurate measurement of insulin dosages because the doses are minute. However, the 1 ml tuberculin syringe or a 3 ml syringe can be used when a U-100 syringe is unavailable.

Dosages measured in units involving oral and parenteral medications

EXAMPLE: Penicillin V 250,000 U p.o. q.i.d. The drug is supplied 200,000 U per 5 ml after reconstitution. Give _____ .

a. On the left side of the proportion, place what you know or have available. In this example each 5 ml contains 200,000 U. So the left side of the proportion would be:

$$200,000 \text{ U}:5 \text{ ml}::$$

b. The right side of the proportion is determined by the physician's order and the abbreviations on the left side of the proportion. Only two different abbreviations may be used in a single proportion. The abbreviations must be in the same position on the right side as on the left side.

$$200,000 \text{ U}:5 \text{ ml}::250,000 \text{ U}: _____ \text{ ml}$$

Since we need to find the number of milliliters to be administered, we use the symbol x to represent the unknown.

$$200,000 \text{ U}:5 \text{ ml}::250,000 \text{ U}:x \text{ ml}$$

c. Rewrite the proportion without using the abbreviations

$$200,000:5::250,000:x$$

d. Solve for x

$$200,000:5::250,000:x$$

$$200,000 \, x = 250,000 \times 5$$

$$200,000x = 1,250,000$$

$$x = \frac{1,250,000}{200,000}$$

$$x = 6.25$$

e. Label your answer as determined by the abbreviation placed next to x in the original proportion.

$$x = 6.25 \text{ ml}$$

6.25 ml would be measured to administer 250,000 U of penicillin V.

Dosages measured in units involving parenteral medications

EXAMPLE: Heparin 12,000 U subq. q. 8 h. Heparin 10,000 U per ml is supplied. Give _____ .

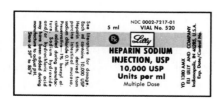

a. 10,000 U:1 ml::

b. 10,000 U:1 ml:: _____ U: _____ ml

10,000 U:1 ml::12,000 U:x ml.

c. $10,000:1::12,000:x$

d. $10,000x = 1 \times 12,000$

$10,000x = 12,000$

$x = \dfrac{12000}{10000}$

$x = 1.2$

e. $x = 1.2$ ml

Therefore 1.2 ml of heparin would be the amount of each individual dose of heparin given q. 8 h.

Insulin given with an insulin low-dose syringe

EXAMPLE: Lente insulin 36 U subq. in A.M. Lente insulin U-100 and a U-100 low-dose syringe are available. Draw a vertical line through the syringe to indicate the correct dosage.

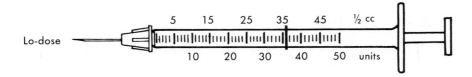

With a low-dose insulin syringe, 36 U of U-100 insulin would be measured as indicated.

Regular insulin given with another type of insulin in the same U-100 syringe

EXAMPLE: Lente humulin insulin 46 U subq. q. A.M. Regular humulin insulin 20 U. Lente humulin insulin U-100, regular humulin insulin U-100, and a U-100 insulin syringe are available. Draw a vertical line through the syringe to indicate the amount of lente humulin insulin to be given, and a second line to indicate the total dosage.

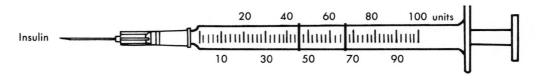

The lente humulin insulin dosage is indicated at 46 U. Add 20 U of regular humulin insulin for a total dosage of 66 U of insulin.

Insulin given with a 1 ml tuberculin syringe

EXAMPLE: NPH insulin 42 U subq. q. A.M. NPH insulin U-100 and a 1 ml tuberculin syringe are available. Give _____ .

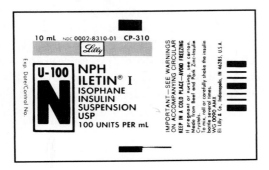

a. 100 U:1 ml::

b. 100 U:1 ml:: _____ U: _____ ml

   100 U:1 ml::42 U:x ml

c. 100:1::42:x

d. 100x = 42

$$x = \frac{42}{100}$$

$$x = 0.42 \text{ ml}$$

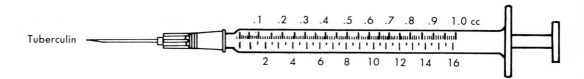

Tuberculin

Insulin given with a 3 ml syringe

EXAMPLE: Lente humulin insulin 48 U subq. q. A.M. Lente humulin insulin U-100 and a 3 ml syringe are available. Give _____ ℳ.

a. 100 U:1 ml::

b. 100 U:1 ml:: _____ U: _____ ml

   100 U:1 ml::48 U:x ml

c. 100:1::48:x

d. 100x = 48

$$x = \frac{48}{100}$$

$$x = 0.48 \text{ ml}$$

a. 15 ℳ:1 ml::

b. 15 ℳ:1 ml:: _____ ℳ: _____ ml

   15 ℳ:1ml::x ℳ:0.48 ml

c. 15:1::x:0.48

   $x = 15 \times 0.48$

   $x = 7.2$ ℳ

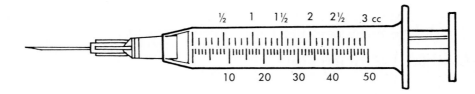

Complete the following work sheet, which provides for extensive practice in the calculation of dosages measured in units. Check your answers. If you have difficulties, go back and review the necessary material. When you feel ready to evaluate your learning, take the first posttest. Check your answers. An acceptable score as indicated on the posttest signifies that you have successfully completed this chapter. An unacceptable score signifies a need for further study before taking the second posttest.

WORK SHEET

The medication order is listed at the beginning of each problem. Calculate the dosages measured in units by the use of a proportion. Show your work.

1. Penicillin V 200,000 U p.o. q.i.d. You have penicillin V oral solution 400,000 U per 5 ml. Give _____ .

2. Heparin 7500 U subq. q. 12 h. Heparin 5000 U per ml is available. Give _____ .

3. NPH insulin 20 U subq. on Tuesday and Thursday A.M. You have a 10 ml vial of NPH insulin U-100 and a 3 ml syringe. Give _____ ℳ.

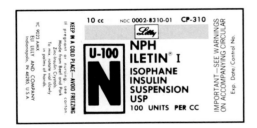

4. Penicillin G 500,000 U I.M. q. 6 h. Penicillin G 1,000,000 U per ml is supplied. Give _____ .

5. Heparin 2500 U, subq. q. 12 h. You have heparin 5000 U per ml. Give _____ .

6. Regular humulin insulin 2 U subq. q. P.M. You have regular humulin insulin U-100 and a U-100 low-dose syringe. Draw a vertical line through the syringe to indicate the dosage.

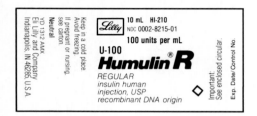

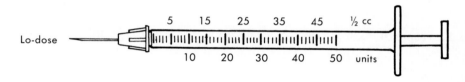

Lo-dose

7. Heparin 5,000 U subq. q. 8 h. You have heparin 10,000 U per ml. Give _____ .

8. V-Cillin K suspension 400,000 U p.o. q. 6 h. V-Cillin K suspension is supplied 200,000 U per 5 ml. Give _____ .

9. Lente insulin 14 U, Regular insulin 6 U subq. q. A.M. Lente insulin U-100, regular insulin U-100, and a U-100 low-dose syringe are supplied. Draw a vertical line through the syringe to indicate the amount of lente insulin to be given, and a second line to indicate the total dosage.

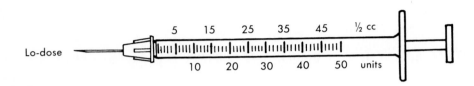

10. Penicillin V 300,000 U p.o. q.i.d. You have penicillin V oral solution 400,000 U per 5 ml. How many ml will you give? _____ .

11. Heparin 6000 U subq. q.d. The drug is supplied 5000 U per ml. Give _____ .

12. Regular insulin 18 U subq. q. A.M. You have regular insulin U-100 and a U-100 low-dose syringe. Draw a vertical line through the syringe to indicate the dosage.

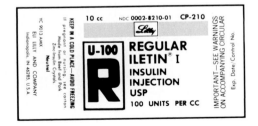

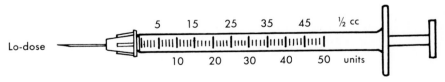

13. NPH insulin 32 U subq. tomorrow at 7:45 A.M. You have NPH insulin U-100 and a tuberculin syringe. Give _____ ml.

14. Penicillin G 600,000 U I.M. b.i.d. You have Penicillin G 1,000,000 U per ml available. Give _____ .

15. Heparin 10,000 U subq. q. 12 h. You have heparin 5000 U per ml. Give _____ .

Answers on p. 359.

Name _____

Date _____

ACCEPTABLE SCORE ____7____

YOUR SCORE _____

POSTTEST 1

DIRECTIONS: The medication order is listed at the beginning of each problem. Calculate the dosages measured in units by the use of a proportion. Show your work.

1. Penicillin V 500,000 U p.o. q.i.d. Penicillin V pediatric suspension 400,000 U per 5 ml is available. Give _____ .

2. Lente insulin 40 U subq. q. A.M. Lente insulin U-100 and a 3 ml syringe are available. Give _____ .

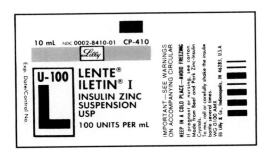

3. Heparin 7500 U subq. q.i.d. You have heparin 5000 U per ml. Give _____ .

4. Regular humulin insulin 6 U subq. Regular humulin insulin and a U-100 syringe are available. Draw a vertical line through the syringe to indicate the dosage.

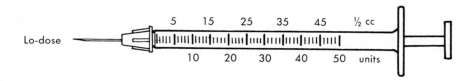

Lo-dose

5. Pfizerpen 3,000,000 U I.M. q. 6 h. Pfizerpen is supplied in a vial containing 1,000,000 U per ml. Give _____ .

6. NPH insulin 40 U subq. q. A.M. You have NPH insulin U-100 and a tuberculin syringe. Give _____ .

7. Heparin 20,000 U subq. today. Heparin 10,000 U per ml is available. Give _____ .

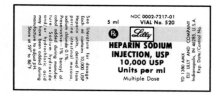

8. Lente insulin 38 U, regular insulin 18 U subq. q. A.M. Lente insulin U-100, regular insulin U-100, and a U-100 syringe are supplied. Draw a vertical line through the syringe to indicate the amount of lente insulin to be given, and a second line to indicate the total dosage.

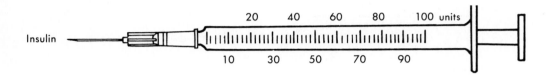

Answers on pp. 359-360.

Name _____

Date _____

ACCEPTABLE SCORE ____7____

YOUR SCORE _____

POSTTEST 2

DIRECTIONS: The medication order is listed at the beginning of each problem. Calculate the
dosages measured in units by the use of a proportion. Show your work.

1. Regular insulin 10 U subq. tomorrow A.M. Regular insulin U-100 and a U-100 low-dose syringe are supplied. Draw a vertical line through the syringe to indicate the dosage.

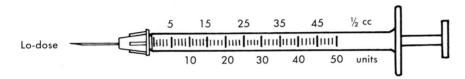

2. Heparin 1000 U per L to be added to I.V. fluids. You have heparin 10,000 U per ml. How
many minims would you add to 1 L? _____ .

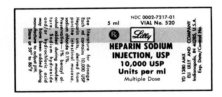

3. V-Cillin K 500,000 U p.o. q. 6 h. You have 200,000 U per ℥ available. Give _____ ℥.

4. NPH insulin 28 U subq. Tuesday and Thursday at 7:45 A.M. You have NPH insulin U-100
and a tuberculin syringe. Give _____ ml.

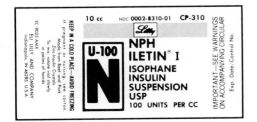

5. Heparin 1500 U subq. today. The drug is supplied 1000 U per ml. Give _____ .

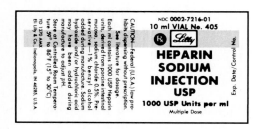

6. Penicillin G potassium 1.2 million U IV. q. 4 h. You have a vial containing 1,000,000 U per ml. Give _____ .

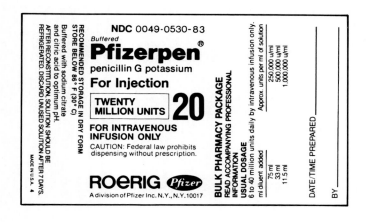

7. Lente insulin 34 U subq. q. A.M. You have lente insulin U-100 and a 3 ml syringe. Give _____ ɱ.

8. NPH insulin 16 U, regular insulin 8 U subq. q. A.M. You have NPH insulin U-100, regular insulin U-100, and a U-100 low-dose syringe. Draw a vertical line through the syringe to indicate the amount of NPH insulin to be given, and a second line to indicate the total dosage.

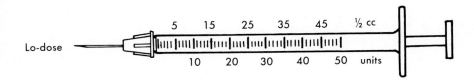

Answers on p. 360.

Name _____

Date _____

ACCEPTABLE SCORE ___14___

YOUR SCORE _____

PRETEST

DIRECTIONS: The intravenous fluid order is listed at the beginning of each problem. Calculate the following IV flow rates by the use of a proportion using the indicated drop factor. Show your work. Place your answers in the space provided and label.

1. Dextra 12% 1000 ml within 10 h. How many ml/h.? _____ . How many ml/min? _____ . How many gtt/min? _____ .
   (drop factor 15)

2. 250 ml N.S. within 12 h. How many ml/h.? _____ . How many ml/min? _____ . How many gtt/min? _____ .
   (drop factor 60)

3. Intralipids 20% 500 ml I.V. within 12 h. M.W.F. Begin today. How many ml/h.? _____ . How many ml/min? _____ . How many gtt/min? _____ .
   (drop factor 12)

4. N.S. at 250 ml/h. today. How many ml/h? _____ . How many ml/min? _____ . How many gutt/min? _____ .
   (drop factor 10)

5. D$_{10}$W 0.25 L within 8 h. How many ml/h.? _____ . How many ml/min? _____ . How many gtt/min? _____ .
   (drop factor 20)

6. 0.9% N.S. 500 ml with 100 U regular insulin. Infuse at 2 U/h. Amount of drug/ml _____ . How many ml/h?_____ . How many ml/min? _____ . How many gtt/min? _____ .
   (drop factor 60)

7. D$_5$W 250 ml with 50,000 U heparin? Infuse at 1200 U/h. Amount of drug/ml _____ . How many ml/h.?_____ . How many ml/min? _____ . How many gtt/min? _____ .
   (drop factor 60)

8. Dobutrex 1 Gm in 250 ml D_5 ½ N.S. Infuse at 15 μg/kg/min for patient weighing 55 kg. Amount of drug/min for 55 kg patient _____ . Amount of drug/ml _____ . How many ml/min? _____ . How many gtt/min? _____ .

    (drop factor 60)

Answers on p. 360.

CHAPTER 13

INTRAVENOUS FLOW RATES

Learning objectives

On completion of the materials provided in this chapter, you will be able to perform computations accurately by mastering the following mathematical concepts:

1. Calculate ml/h. of I.V. flow rates when total volume and length of time over which the I.V. is to infuse is given
2. Calculate ml/min of I.V flow rates when total volume and length of time over which the I.V. is to infuse is given
3. Calculate gtt/min if I.V. flow rates when total volume and length of time over which the I.V. is to infuse is given
4. Calculate ml/min of I.V. flow rates when ml/h. is given
5. Calculate gtt/min of I.V. flow rates when ml/h. is given

It is sometimes necessary to deliver fluids and medications to a patient intravenously. Intravenous solutions and medications are placed directly into a vein. Infusions are injections of large quantities of fluids and nutrients into the patient's venous system.

An intravenous medication or infusion may be prepared and administered by the physician, nurse, or technician as regulated by state law and the policies of the particular health care agency. Medications and electrolyte milliequivalents are frequently ordered as additives of I.V. fluids. Medications may also be diluted and given in conjunction with I.V. solutions.

I.V. fluids are administered via an intravenous infusion set. This set includes the sealed bottle or bag containing the fluids, a drip chamber connected to the bottle or bag by a small tube or spike, and tubing that leads from the drip chamber down to and connecting with the needle or catheter at the site of insertion into the patient. The flow rate is adjusted to the desired drops per minute by a clamp placed around the tubing. It is necessary for the nurse to be knowledgeable about the equipment being used and, in particular, about the flow rate or drops per milliliter that a particualr set of tubing will deliver.

Infusion sets come in a variety of sizes. The larger the diameter of the tubing where it enters the drip chamber, the bigger the drop will be. The drop factor of an infusion set is the number of drops contained in 1 ml (1 cc). This equivalent may vary with different manufacturers. The most frequent drop factors are 10, 12, 15, 20, and 60. Sets that deliver 10, 12, 15, or 20 drops per milliliter are know as macrodrip sets. A set that delivers 60 drops per milliliter is know as a microdrip set. The macrodrip sets are larger than the microdrips.

If large volumes of fluid must be administered (125 ml/h or more), a macrodrip set would be required. The microdrip sets are unable to deliver large volumes per hour because their drop size is so small. When the I.V. solution is to run at a rate of 50 ml/h. or less, a microdrip set should be used. Some hospitals may even require a microdrip set for rates of 60 to 80 ml/h., for accuracy of flow rate and to help maintain the patency of the line. The number of drops per milliliter for the I.V. administration set is written on the outside of the box. This is essential information in solving problems related to the regulation of I.V. flow rates.

The physician is responsible for writing the order for the type of intravenous or hyperalimentation fluids and amount. The number of hours or rate of infusion is also ordered by the physician. It is usually the nurse's responsibility to regulate and maintain the infusion flow rate. It is the goal of the nurse to ensure that the I.V. flow be regular. If the rate is irregular, too much or too little fluid may be infused. This may lead to a variety of complications such as fluid overload, dehydration, or medication overdose. Sometimes the rate of flow must be adjusted because of interruptions due to needle placement, condition of the vein, or infiltration.

The nurse must be able to determine the number of drops per minute the patient must receive in order for the infusion to be completed within the specified time. To accomplish this task, the nurse must calculate three different pieces of information in the following manner:

1. Milliliters given per hour (ml/h.)
2. Milliters given per minue (ml/min)
3. Drops given per minute (gtt/min)

All three of these items may be calculated by the use of a proportion.

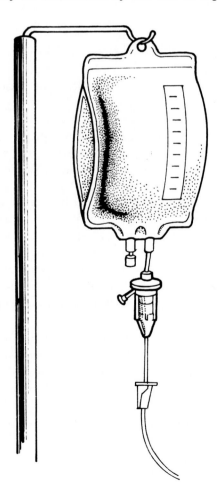

Intravenous
set

EXAMPLE: Amigen 500 ml in 3 h. How many ml must be given per hour? _____ .
How many ml must be given per minute? _____ . How many gtt must be
given per minute? _____ .
   (drop factor 15)

1. ml/h.

$$500 \text{ ml}:3\text{h}.::x \text{ ml}:1 \text{ h}.$$

$$500:3::x:1$$

$$3x = 500$$

$$x = \frac{500}{3}$$

$$x = 166,66 \text{ ml}$$

$$166.66 \text{ ml/h}.$$

2. ml/min

To determine the drops per minute the nurse must first calculate the number of
milliliters the patient must receive per minute. We have already determined
that the patient must receive 166.66 ml per 1 hour, or 60 minutes. Therefore the
following proportion may be written:

$$166.66 \text{ ml}:60 \text{ min}::x \text{ ml}:1 \text{ min}$$

$$166.66:60::x:1$$

$$60x = 166.66$$

$$x = \frac{166.66}{60}$$

$$x = 2.777 \cdots$$

$$x = 2.78 \text{ ml}$$

$$2.78 \text{ ml/min}$$

3. gtt/min

This number and calculation depend on the drop factor of the tubing you are
using. Remember, this information is found on the package. For the problems in
this workbook, the drop factor will be indicated. The drop factor for this problem is 15. We have just determined that the patient must receive 2.78 ml each
minute. Therefore the following proportion may be written:

$$15 \text{ gtt}:1 \text{ ml}::x \text{ gtt}:2.78 \text{ ml}$$

$$15:1::x:2.78$$

$$x = 15 \times 2.78$$

$$x = 41.70$$

$$x = 41.70, \text{ or rounded to } 42 \text{ gtt}$$

The nurse thus knows how to regulate the I.V. to drop at 42 drops per minute,
for the full 500 ml to be infused within the 3 hours ordered.

4. Shortcut

When the volume per hour is known, a different formula may be used by the nurse who has a great deal of mathematical expertise. This formula combines steps 2 and 3.

$$\text{drops per minute} = \frac{\text{volume per hour}}{60 \text{ minutes}} \times \frac{\text{drop factor}}{1}$$

EXAMPLE: We have determined that the hourly rate is 166.66 or 167 ml per hour or 60 minutes. The problem indicates the drop factor is 15. Therefore, the equation would be as follows:

$$x \text{ (gtt/min)} = \frac{167 \text{ (volume per hour)}}{60 \text{ (minutes per hour)}} \times \frac{15 \text{ (drop factor)}}{1}$$

$$x = \frac{167}{\overset{}{\underset{4}{\cancel{60}}}} \times \frac{\overset{1}{\cancel{15}}}{1}$$

$$x = \frac{167}{4}$$

$$x = 41.75, \text{ or rounded to 42 gtt/min}$$

Once again the nurse knows to regulate the I.V. to drip at 42 drops per minute for the full 500 ml to be infused within the 3 hours ordered.

EXAMPLE: 250 ml D$_5$W in 24 h. How many ml will be given per hour? _____ . How many ml/min will be given? _____ . How many gtt will be given per minute? _____ .

(drop factor 60)

1. ml/h.

$$250 \text{ ml} : 24 \text{ h.} :: x \text{ ml} : 1 \text{ h.}$$

$$250 : 24 :: x : 1$$

$$24x = 250$$

$$x = \frac{250}{24}$$

$$x = 10.41 \text{ ml}$$

$$x = 10.41 \text{ ml/h.}$$

2. ml/min

$$10.41 \text{ ml} : 60 \text{ min} :: x : 1 \text{ min}$$

$$10.41 : 60 :: x : 1$$

$$60x = 10.41$$

$$x = \frac{10.41}{60}$$

$$x = 0.17$$

$$x = 0.17 \text{ ml/min}$$

3. gtt/min

$$60 \text{ gtt}:1 \text{ ml}::x \text{ gtt}:0.17 \text{ ml}$$

$$60:1::x:0.17$$

$$x = 60 \times 0.17$$

$$x = 10.2$$

$$x = 10.2 \text{ or } 10 \text{ gtt/min}$$

4. Shortcut

$$x \text{ (gtt/min)} = \frac{10 \text{ (volume per hour)}}{60 \text{ (minutes per hour)}} \times \frac{60 \text{ (drop factor)}}{1}$$

$$x = \frac{10}{\underset{1}{\cancel{60}}} \times \frac{\overset{1}{\cancel{60}}}{1}$$

$$x = 10$$

$$x = 10 \text{ gtt/min}$$

NOTE: When a microdrip set (drop factor of 60) is used, the drops per minute will be the same as the number of milliliters per hour.

Sometimes the physician writes the order for the type of fluid plus the rate at which it is to infuse. In that case only the second and third calculations need to be made.

EXAMPLE: $D_5\frac{1}{2}$ N.S at 120 ml/h. How many ml/min will be given? _____ . How many gtt/min will be given? _____ .
(drop factor 12)

1. 120 ml/h. given in order
2. ml/min

$$120 \text{ ml}:60 \text{ min}::x \text{ ml}:1 \text{ min}$$

$$120:60::x:1$$

$$60x = 120$$

$$x = \frac{120}{60}$$

$$x = 2$$

$$x = 2 \text{ ml/min}$$

3. gtt/min

$$12 \text{ gtt}:1 \text{ ml}::x\text{gtt}:2 \text{ ml}$$

$$12:1::x:2$$

$$x = 24$$

$$x = 24 \text{ gtt/min}$$

4. Shortcut

$$x \text{ (gtt/min)} = \frac{120 \text{ (volume per hour)}}{60 \text{ (minutes per hour)}} \times \frac{12 \text{ (drop factor)}}{1}$$

$$x = \frac{120}{\underset{5}{\cancel{60}}} \times \frac{\overset{1}{\cancel{12}}}{1}$$

$$x = \frac{120}{5}$$

$$x = 24$$

$$x = 24 \text{ gtt/min}$$

Critical care I.V. medications and flow rates

Critically ill patients in the hospital frequently receive special medications that are very potent and therefore need to be monitored closely. Some of these medications may be ordered at a set amount of the drug measured in units to be infused over a given period of time, for example, regular insulin or heparin. Other drugs used in the critical care setting may be ordered infused by amount of drug per kilogram of body weight per minute. These are known as titrations. They are based on the manufacturer's provided recommended dosage and the patient's body weight measured in kilograms. In most health care institutions, these situations will occur only in the emergency room or the intensive care unit. It is extremely important to accurately monitor the flow of these medications; therefore, most are delivered through an I.V. machine. Because of the nature of these drugs, route of administration, and state of the patient, it cannot be overemphasized how important the accuracy of the calculation of the drug dosage and I.V. flow rates is. It is truly a matter of life and death.

This chapter will provide a sampling of these types of calculations. However, to become competent and develop expertise in this area, we would recommend further in-depth study in a clinical setting with experienced supervision.

I.V. administration of regular insulin and heparin

EXAMPLE: 0.9% N.S. 500 ml with 200 U regular insulin. Infuse 10 U/h. Amount of drug/ml _____ . How many ml/h? _____ . How many ml/min? _____ . How many gtt/min? _____ .
(drop factor 60)

1. First determine the amount of drug in each milliliter. This may be done by the use of a proportion.

500 ml N.S.:200 U insulin::1 ml N.S. :x U insulin

$$500:200::1:x$$

$$500x = 200$$

$$x = \frac{200}{500}$$

$$x = 0.4$$

$$x = 0.4 \text{ U insulin/ml}$$

2. ml/h

0.4 U insulin:1 ml::10 U insulin:x ml

$$0.4:1::10:x$$

$$0.4x = 10$$

$$x = \frac{10}{0.4}$$

$$x = 25$$

$$x = 25 \text{ ml/h.}$$

3. ml/min

25 ml:60 min::x:1 min

$$25:60::x:1$$

$$60x = 25$$

$$x = \frac{25}{60}$$

$$x = 0.416$$

$$0.42 \text{ ml/min}$$

4. gtt/min

60 gtt:1 ml::x gtt:0.42 ml

$$60:1::x:0.42$$

$$x = 25.2$$

$$x = 25.2 \text{ gtt/min}$$

5. Shortcut

$$x \text{ (gtt/min)} = \frac{25 \text{ (volume per hour)}}{60 \text{ (minutes per hour)}} \times \frac{60 \text{ (drop factor)}}{1}$$

$$x = \frac{25}{\cancel{60}} \times \frac{\overset{1}{\cancel{60}}}{1}$$

$$x = 25 \text{ gtt/min}$$

EXAMPLE: D_5W 1000 ml with 40,000 U heparin. Infuse at 2000 U/h. Amount of drug/ml _____ . How many ml/h? _____ . How many ml/min? _____ . How many gtt/min? _____ .
  (drop factor 60)

1. Amount of drug/ml

1000 ml D_5W:40,000 U heparin::1 ml D_5W:x U heparin

$$1000:40,000::1:x$$

$$1000x = 40,000$$

$$x = 40$$

$$40 \text{ U heparin/ml}$$

2. ml/h

40 U heparin:1 ml D$_5$W::2000 U heparin:x ml D$_5$W

$$40:1::2000:x$$

$$40x = 2000$$

$$x = 50$$

50 ml/h.

3. ml/min

50 ml:60 min::x ml:1 min

$$50:60::x:1$$

$$60x = 50$$

$$x = 0.833$$

0.83 ml/min

4. gtt/min

60 gtt:1 ml::x:0.83 ml

$$60:1::x:0.83$$

$$x = 49.8$$

$$x = 49.8 \text{ gtt/min}$$

5. Shortcut

$$x \text{ (gtt/min)} = \frac{50 \text{ (volume per hour)}}{60 \text{ (minutes per hour)}} \times \frac{60 \text{ (drop factor)}}{1}$$

$$x = \frac{50}{\cancel{60}} \times \frac{\overset{1}{\cancel{60}}}{1}$$

$$x = 50 \text{ gtt/min}$$

I.V. administration of medication per kilogram per minute

EXAMPLE: Dopamine 1 Gm in 250 ml D$_5$ ½ N.S. Infuse at 3 µg/kg/min for a patient weighing 65 kg. Amount of drug/min for 65 kg patient _____ . Amount of drug/ml _____ . How many ml/min? _____ . How many gtt/min? _____ . *(drop factor 60)*

1. Amount of drug per minute for 65 kg patient

3 µg:1 kg::x µg:65 kg

$$3:1::x:65$$

$$x = 195$$

195 µg/min for this 65 kg patient

2. Amount of drug/ml
Since the order is in micrograms, change 1 Gm to micrograms. (Refer to Chapter 7.) You should know that 1 Gm equals 1,000,000 µg. To find the amount of drug in each milliliter, use the following proportion:

$$1{,}000{,}000 \ \mu g : 250 \ ml :: x \ \mu g : 1 \ ml$$

$$1{,}000{,}000 : 250 :: x : 1$$

$$250 \ x = 1{,}000{,}000$$

$$x = \frac{1{,}000{,}000}{250}$$

$$x = 4000$$

$$4000 \ \mu g/ml$$

3. ml/min

$$4000 \ \mu g : 1 \ ml :: 195 \ \mu g : x \ ml$$

$$4000 : 1 :: 19 : x$$

$$4000x = 195$$

$$x = \frac{195}{4000}$$

$$x = 0.048 \ ml$$

0.048 ml/min must be infused for this 65 kg patient

4. gtt/min

$$60 \ gtt : 1 \ ml :: x \ gtt : 0.048 \ ml$$

$$60 : 1 :: x : 0.048$$

$$x = 2.88$$

$$x = 2.88 \ or \ 3 \ gtt/min$$

Complete the following work sheet, which provides for extensive practice in the calculation if I.V. flow rates. Check your answers. If you have difficulties, go back and review the necessary material. When you feel ready to evaluate your learning, take the first posttest. Check your answers. An acceptable score as indicated on the posttest signifies that you have successfully completed this chapter. An unacceptable score signifies a need for further study before taking the second posttest.

WORK SHEET

The I.V. fluid order is listed at the beginning of each problem. Calculate the following I.V. flow rates by the use of a proportion, using the indicated drop factor. Show your work. Place your answers in the space provided and label.

1. Dextran 12% 1000 ml within 8 h. How many ml/h.? _____ . How many ml/min? _____ . How many gtt/min? _____ .
   (drop factor 12)

2. Amigen 800 ml within 8 h. How many ml/h.? _____ . How many ml/min? _____ . How many gtt/min? _____ .
   (drop factor 10)

3. Cytoxan 475 mg in 250 ml D_5W over 2 h. How many ml/h.? _____ . How many ml/min? _____ . How many gtt/min? _____ .
   (drop factor 15)

4. 1.5 L of 5% glucoe in DW within 10 h. How many ml/h? _____ . How many ml/min? _____ . How many gtt/min? _____ .
 (drop factor 15)

5. N.S. Sol. 3000 ml within 48 h. How many ml/h? _____ . How many ml/min? _____ . How many gtt/min? _____ .
 (drop factor 10)

6. 1000 ml D_5W c̄ 100 mEq KCl to infuse at 100 ml/h. How many ml/h? _____ . How many ml/min? _____ . How many gtt/min? _____ .
 (drop factor 12)

7. Blood plasma 500 ml within 4 h. How many ml/h? _____ . How many ml/min? _____ . How many gtt/min? _____ .
 (drop factor 15)

8. Ringer's lactate 1500 ml within 16 h. How many ml/h? _____ . How many ml/min? _____ . How many gtt/min? _____ .
 (drop factor 10)

DIRECTIONS: Use the shortcut method to determine the gtt/min in problems 9 through 12.

9. $D_{10}\frac{1}{4}$ N.S. $\bar{c}$ 20 mEq KCl + 1000 U heparin/L at 10 ml/h. How many ml/h.? _____ . How many ml/min? _____ . How many gtt/min? _____ .
   (drop factor 60)

10. Packed red blood cells 1 U (0.5 L) within 6 h. How many ml/h.? _____ . How many ml/min? _____ . How many gtt/min? _____ .
   (drop factor 12)

11. Multiple electrolytes 0.8 L within 6 h. How many ml/h.? _____ . How many ml/min? _____ . How many gtt/min? _____ .
   (drop factor 15)

12. D_{10}W 250 ml + 7.5 mEq NaCl + 5.0 mEq KCl at 2 ml/h. How many ml/h.? _____ . How many ml/min? _____ . How many gtt/min? _____ .
   (drop factor 60)

13. 0.9% N.S. 250 ml with 100 U regular insulin. Infuse at 12 U/h. Amount of drug/ml _____ . How many ml/h.? _____ . How many ml/min? _____ . How many gtt/min? _____ .
   (drop factor 60)

14. 0.9% N.S. 500 ml with 100 U regular insulin. Infuse at 8 U/h. Amount of drug/ml _____ . How many ml/h.? _____ . How many ml/min? _____ . How many gtt/min? _____ .
  (drop factor 60)

15. D$_5$W 500 ml with 10,000 U heparin. Infuse at 100 U/h. Amount of drug/ml _____ . How many ml/h.? _____ . How many ml/min? _____ . How many gtt/min? _____ .
  (drop factor 60)

16. 0.9% N.S. 1000 ml with 30,000 U heparin. Infuse at 1000 U/h. Amount of drug/ml _____ . How many ml/h.? _____ . How many ml/min? _____ . How many gtt/min? _____ .
  (drop factor 60)

17. Dobutamine 1 Gm in 250 ml D$_5$ ½ N.S. Infuse at 12 μg/kg/min for a patient weighing 75 kg. Amount of drug/min for 75 kg patient _____ . Amount of drug/ml _____ . How many ml/min? _____ . How many gtt/min? _____ .
  (drop factor 60)

18. Aminophylline 2 Gm in 1000 ml D$_5$W. Infuse at 0.4 mg/kg/h. for a patient weighing 55 kg. Amount of drug/min for 55 kg patient _____ . Amount of drug/ml _____ . How many ml/min? _____ . How many gtt/min? _____ .
  (drop factor 60)

19. Nitroglycerin 100 mg in 500 ml D$_5$W. Infuse at 3 μg/kg/min for patient weighing 66 kg. Amount of drug/min for 66 kg patient _____ . Amount of drug/ml _____ . How many ml/min? _____ . How many gtt/min? _____ .
   (drop factor 60)

20. Dobutamine 250 mg in 250 ml D$_5$W. Infuse at 50 μg/kg/min for patient weighing 80 kg. Amount of drug/min for 80 kg patient _____ . Amount of drug/ml _____ . How many ml/min? _____ . How many gtt/min? _____ .
   (drop factor 60)

Answers on p. 360.

Name _____

Date _____

ACCEPTABLE SCORE ___13___

YOUR SCORE _____

POSTTEST 1

DIRECTIONS: The I.V. fluid order is listed at the beginning of each problem. Calculate the following I.V. flow rates by the use of a proportion using the indicated drop factor. Show your work. Place your answers in the space provided and label.

1. Ringer's lactate 1000 ml within 12 h. How many ml/h? _____. How many ml/min? _____. How many gtt/min? _____.
   (drop factor 15)

2. Blood plasma 0.5 L in 4 h. How many ml/h? _____. How many ml/min? _____. How many gtt/min? _____.
   (drop factor 12)

3. N.S. to infuse at 150 ml/h. How many ml/h? _____. How many ml/min? _____. How many gtt/min? _____.
   (drop factor 15)

4. $D_{10}W$ 750 ml in 10 h. How many ml/h? _____. How many ml/min? _____. How many gtt/min? _____.
   (drop factor 10)

5. Otic 150 mg in 50 ml D₅W over 30 min. How many ml/min? _____ . How many gtt/min? _____ .

    (drop factor 12)

6. 0.9% N.S. 1000 ml with 500 U regular insulin. Infuse at 9 U/h. Amount of drug/ml _____ . How many ml/h? _____ . How many ml/min? _____ . How many gtt/min? _____ .
    (drop factor 60)

7. D₅W 1000 ml with 30,000 U heparin. Infuse at 500 U/h. Amount of drug/ml _____ . How many ml/h? _____ . How many ml/min? _____ . How many gtt/min? _____ .
    (drop factor 60)

8. Nipride 50 mg in 250 ml D₅W. Infuse at 3 μg/kg/min for patient weighing 82 kg. Amount of drug/min for 82 kg patient _____ . Amount of drug/ml _____ . How many ml/min? _____ . How many gtt/min? _____ .
    (drop factor 60)

Answers on p. 360

Name _____

Date _____

ACCEPTABLE SCORE ___14___

YOUR SCORE _____

POSTTEST 2

DIRECTIONS: The intravenous fluid order is listed at the beginning of each problem. Calculate the following IV flow rates by the use of a proportion using the indicated drop factor. Show your work. Place your answers in the space provided and label.

1. Whole blood 500 ml within 6 h. How many ml/h? _____ . How many ml/min? _____ .
How many gtt/min? _____ .
(drop factor 15)

2. $D_5\frac{1}{2}$N.S with 20 mEq KCl/L at 30 ml/h. How many ml/h? _____ . How many ml/min?
_____ . How many gtt/min? _____ .
(drop factor 20)

3. 5% glucose in N.S. 1000 ml, followed by 1000 ml D_5W, followed by N.S 1000 ml within 24 h.
How many ml/h? _____ . How many ml/min? _____ . How many gtt/min? _____ .
(drop factor 12)

4. D_5W 250 ml at 3 ml/h. How many ml/h? _____ . How many ml/min? _____ . How many
gtt/min? _____ .
(drop factor 60)

5. ½ N.S. 1000 ml within 18 h. How many ml/h? _____ . How many ml/min? _____ . How many gtt/min? _____

    (drop factor 10)

6. 0.9% N.S. 250 ml with 250 U regular insulin. Infuse at 7 U/h. Amount of drug/ml _____ . How many ml/h? _____ . How many ml/min? _____ . How many gtt/min? _____ .

    (drop factor 60)

7. D$_5$W 1000 ml with 30,000 U heparin. Infuse at 1500 U/h. Amount of drug/ml _____ . How many ml/h? _____ . How many ml/min? _____ . How many gtt/min? _____ .

    (drop factor 60)

8. Neo-Synephrine 10 mg in 500 ml D$_5$W. Infuse at 0.5 µg/kg/min for patient weighing 75 kg. Amount of drug/min for 75 kg patient _____ . Amount of drug/ml _____ . How many ml/min? _____ . How many gtt/min? _____ .

    (drop factor 60)

Answers on p. 360.

Name _____

Date _____

ACCEPTABLE SCORE ____4____

YOUR SCORE _____

PRETEST

DIRECTIONS: The medication order is listed at the beginning of each problem. Calculate the child's weight in kilograms, determine the safe recommended dosage or range, determine the safety of the order, and calculate the drug dosage by the use of a proportion. Show your work. Place the answer in the spaces provided and label.

1. Erythromycin 100 mg p.o. q.6 h. for a child weighing 24 lbs. You have erythromycin 199 mg/ml. The recommended daily p.o. dose for a child is 30 to 50 mg/kg/day in divided dosages q.8 h. Child's weight is _____ kg. Safe recommended dose or range for this child is _____ . Is the order safe? _____ . If yes, give _____ .

2. Tobramycin sulfate 15 mg I.M. q.6 h. for a child weighing 22 lbs. Tobramycin 10 mg/ml is available. The recommended daily I.M. dosage for a child is 6 to 7.5 mg/kg/day in equally divided dosages q.6 h. Child's weight is _____ kg. Safe recommended dosage or range for this child is _____ . Is the order safe? _____ . If yes, give _____ .

3. Prednisone 10 mg p.o. q.i.d. for a child weighing 88 lbs. You have prednisone 2.5 mg tablets. The recommended daily p.o. dose for a child is 0.14 to 2 mg/kg/day in divided dosages q.i.d. Child's weight is _____ kg. Safe recommended dosage or range for this child is _____ . Is the order safe? _____ . If yes, give _____ .

4. Demerol 50 mg I.M. 1 hour before surgery for a child weighing 52 lb. Demerol 50 mg/ml is available. The recommended daily I.M. dose for a child is 1 to 2.2 mg/kg. Child's weight is _____ kg. The safe recommended dosage or range for this child is _____. Is the order safe? _____ . If yes, give _____.

5. Aminophylline 25 mg p.o. q.8 h. for a child weighing 35 lb. You have aminophylline 105 mg/5 ml. The recommended daily p.o. dosage for a child is 3 to 6 mg/kg/day in divided dosages q.8 h. Child's weight is _____ kg. Safe recommended dosage or range for this child is _____ . Is the order safe? _____ . If yes, give _____.

Answers on p. 361.

CHAPTER 14
PEDIATRIC DOSAGES

Learning objectives

On completion of the materials provided in this chapter, you will be able to perform computations accurately by mastering the following mathematical concepts:

1. Convert the weight of the child from pounds to kilograms
2. Use a formula based on body weight to determine the correct dosage of a medication to be administered to a child

Because of their age, weight, height, and physical condition, children are more sensitive to medications than adults. Therefore careful attention must be given when preparing and administering medications to children. The right amount of the right medication must be given to the right child at the right time, in the right way.

Although the physician prescribes the medication, the nurse who administers the medication is responsible for errors in the calculation of the dosage and in the preparation and administration of the drug. The medication order must be accurate—a dosage that is too high may be unsafe and a dosage that is too low may not have the desired therapeutic effect.

To be sure the dosage is within a safe range for the child, we will use the most accurate method of calculating children's dosages, which is the amount of the drug in relation to the child's weight in kilograms for a 24-hour period.

Pediatric dosages calculated by mg/kg/hr

EXAMPLE: Amoxicillin 125 mg p.o. t.i.d. for a child weighing 34.32 lb. You have amoxicillin suspension 125 mg/5 ml. The recommended daily p.o. dose for a child is 20 to 40 mg/kg/day in divided dosages q.8 h. Child's weight is _____ kg. Safe recommended dosage or range for this child is_____ . Is the order safe? _____ . If yes, give _____.

a. Change child's weight to kg (refer to Chapter 8).

$$2.2 \text{ lb} : 1 \text{ kg} :: 34.32 \text{ lb} : x \text{ kg}$$

$$2.2 : 1 :: 34.32 : x$$

$$2.2x = 34.32$$

$$x = \frac{34.32}{2.2}$$

$$x = 15.6 \text{ kg}$$

b. Write a proportion(s) using the recommended dosage and child's weight as your known values to determine the safe recommended dosage or range for this child.

$$20 \text{ mg} : 1 \text{ kg} :: x \text{ mg} : 15.6 \text{ kg}$$

$$20 : 1 :: x : 15.6$$

$$x = 312 \text{ mg}$$

$$40 \text{ mg} : 1 \text{ kg} :: x \text{ mg} : 15.6 \text{ kg}$$

$$40 : 1 :: x : 15.6$$

$$x = 624 \text{ mg}$$

The safe recommended range for this child, who weighs 15.6 kg, is 312 to 624 mg in a 24 hour period.

c. Determine total amount of medication ordered per 24-hour period.

$$125 \text{ mg} : 1 \text{ dose} :: x \text{ mg} : 3 \text{ doses}$$

$$125 : 1 :: x : 3$$

$$x = 375 \text{ mg/ 24 h. period}$$

The order is safe since it falls within the recommended 24-hour range of 312 to 624 mg for this medication and this child.

d. Calculate the actual dosage amount to be given by the use of a proportion (refer to Chapter 10).

$$125 \text{ mg} : 5 \text{ ml} :: 125 \text{ mg} : x \text{ ml}$$

$$125 : 5 :: 125 : x$$

$$125x = 625$$

$$x = 5 \text{ ml}$$

Therefore 5 ml is the amount of each individual t.i.d. dose.

Complete the following work sheet, which provides for extensive practice in the calculation of pediatric dosages. Check your answers. If you have difficulties, go back and review the necessary material. When you feel ready to evaluate your learning, take the first posttest. Check your answers. An acceptable score as indicated on the posttest signifies that you have successfully completed this chapter. An unacceptable score signifies a need for further study before taking the second posttest.

CHAPTER 14
PEDIATRIC DOSAGES

WORK SHEET

DIRECTIONS: The medication order is listed at the beginning of each problem. Calculate the child's weight in kilograms, determine the safe recommended dosage or range, determine the safety of the order, and calculate the drug dosage using a proportion. Show your work. Place the answer in the spaces provided and label.

1. Ceclor 250 mg p.o. t.i.d. for a child weighing 50 lb. You have Ceclor 250 mg capsules. The recommended daily p.o. dose for a child is 20 to 40 mg/kg/day in divided doses q.8 h. Child's weight is _____ kg. Safe recommended dose or range for this child is _____ . Is the order safe? _____ . If yes, give _____.

2. Lanoxin 12.5 mg p.o. q.d. for an infant weighing 6½ lb. You have Lanoxin 0.05 mg/ml. The recommended daily dose for an infant is 0.035 to 0.06 mg/kg/day in divided doses q.8 h. Child's weight is _____ kg. Safe recommended dose or range for this child is _____ . Is the order safe? _____ . If yes, give _____.

3. Benadryl 25 mg I.V. q.6 h. for a child weighing 50 lb. You have Benadryl 10 mg/ml. The recommended daily dose for a child greater than 12 kg is 5 mg/kg/day in four divided doses. Child's weight is _____ kg. Safe recommended dose or range for this child is _____ . Is the order safe? _____ . If yes, give _____.

4. Thorazine 10 mg I.V. q.6 h. for a child weighing 44 lb. You have Thorazine 25 mg/ml. The recommended daily dose is 0.55 mg/kg/q.6 to 8 h. Child's weight is _____ kg. Safe recommended dose or range for this child is _____ . Is the order safe? _____ . If yes, give _____ .

5. Thioguanine 60 mg p.o. today for a child weighing 78 lb. You have Thioguanine 40 mg tablets. The recommended p.o. dose is 2 mg/kg/day. Child's weight is _____ kg. Safe recommended dose or range for this child is _____ . Is the order safe? _____ . If yes, give _____ .

6. Initial dose of Lasix 10 mg p.o. q.d. for a child weighing 30.31 lb. You have Lasix 10 mg/ml. The recommended p.o. dose is 2 mg/kg/day. Child's weight is _____ kg. Safe recommended dose or range for this child is _____ . Is the order safe? _____ . If yes, give _____ .

7. Theophylline 16 mg p.o. q.6 h. for a child weighing 28 lb. You have theophylline elixir 11.25 mg/ml. The recommended p.o. dose should not exceed 12 mg/kg/24 h. Child's weight is _____ kg. Safe recommended dose or range for this child is _____ . Is the order safe? _____ . If yes, give _____ .

8. Dilantin 75 mg p.o. q.12 h. for a child weighing 66 lb. You have Dilantin chewable 50 mg tablets. The recommended p.o. dose for a child is 5 to 7 mg/kg/day in divided doses q. 12 h. Child's weight is _____ kg. Safe recommended dose or range for this child is _____ . Is the order safe? _____ . If yes, give _____.

Answers on p. 361.

Name _____

Date _____

ACCEPTABLE SCORE ____4____

YOUR SCORE _____

POSTTEST 1

DIRECTIONS: The medication order is listed at the beginning of each problem. Calculate the child's weight in kilograms, determine the safe recommended dosage or range, determine the safety of the order, and calculate the drug dosage by the use of a proportion. Show your work. Place the answer in the spaces provided and label.

1. Phenobarbital 60 mg p.o. q.12 h. for a child weighing 55 lb. Elixir of phenobarbital 20 mg/5 ml is available. The recommended daily dose for a child is 4 to 6 mg/kg/day in divided dosages q. 12 h. Child's weight is _____ kg. Safe recommended dosage or range for this child is _____ . Is the order safe? _____ . If yes, give _____ .

2. Lincocin 500 mg p.o. q.6 h. for a child weighing 44 lb. Lincocin is supplied in 250 mg capsules. The recommended daily p.o. dose for a child is 30 to 60 mg/kg/day in divided dosages q.6 h. Child's weight is _____ kg. Safe recommended dosage or range for this child is _____ . Is the order safe? _____ . If yes, give _____ .

3. Procaine penicillin G 150,000 U I.M. q.12 h. for a child weighing 6¾ lb. You have procaine penicillin G 300,000 U/ml. The recommended daily I.M. dosage for a child is 50,000 U q.d. Child's weight is _____ kg. Safe recommended dosage or range for this child is _____ . Is the order safe? _____ . If yes, give _____ .

4. Ceclor 250 mg p.o. t.i.d. for a child weighing 44 lb. Ceclor is supplied in 125 mg/5 ml. The recommended daily p.o. dosage for a child is 20 to 40 mg/kg/day in divided dosages q.8 h. Child's weight is _____ kg. Safe recommended dosage or range for this child is _____ . Is the order safe? _____ . If so, give _____ .

5. Morphine 4 mg I.M. STAT for a child weighing 78 lb. You have morphine sulfate 50 mg/ml. The recommended I.M. dosage for a child is 0.1 to 0.2 mg/kg/day.
Child's weight is _____ kg. Safe recommended dosage for this child is _____ .
Is the order safe? _____ . If yes, give _____ .

Answers on p. 361.

Name _____

Date _____

ACCEPTABLE SCORE ___4___

YOUR SCORE _____

POSTTEST 2

DIRECTIONS: The medication order is listed at the beginning of each problem. Calculate the child's weight in kilograms, determine the safe recommended dosage or range, determine the safety of the order, and calculate the drug dosage by the use of a proportion. Show your work. Place the answer in the spaces provided and label.

1. Cleocin 225 mg I.V. q.6 h. for a child weighing 58 lb. You have Cleocin 150 mg/ml. The recommended daily dosage for a child is 15 to 40 mg/kg/day in divided dosages q. 6-8 h. Child's weight is _____ kg. Safe recommended dosage or range for this child is _____ . Is the order safe? _____ . If yes, give _____ .

2. Dilantin 50 mg p.o. q.12 h. for a child weighing 70 lb. You have Dilantin 30 mg/5 ml. The recommended daily p.o. dosage for a child is 5 to 7 mg/kg in divided dosages q.12 h. Child's weight is _____ kg. Safe recommended dosages or range for this child is _____ . Is the order safe? _____ . If yes, give _____ .

3. Amoxil 250 mg p.o. q.8 h. for a child weighing 58 lb. You have Amoxil 125 mg/5 ml. The recommended daily p.o. dosage for the child is 20 to 40 mg/kg/day in divided dosages q.8 h. Child's weight is _____ kg. Safe recommended dosage or range for this child is _____ . Is the order safe? _____ . If yes, give _____ .

4. Keflex 500 mg p.o. q.6 h. for a child weighing 99 lb. You have Keflex 250 mg capsules available. The recommended daily p.o. dose for a child is 25 to 50 mg/kg/day in four equal dosages q.6 h. Child's weight is _____ kg. Safe recommended dosage or range for this child is _____ . Is the order safe? _____ . If yes, give _____ .

5. Cloxacillin 500 mg p.o. q.6 h. for a child weighing 66 lb. You have Cloxacillin 125 mg/ml available. The recommended daily p.o. dose for a child is 50 to 100 mg/kg in divided dosages q.6 h. Child's weight is _____ kg. Safe recommended dosage or range for this child is _____ . Is the order safe? _____ . If yes, give _____ .

Answers on p. 361.

CHAPTER 15

SPECIAL CONSIDERATIONS FOR THE ELDERLY

People are living longer than at any period in history, and we know more about protecting health and preventing illness. By practicing good health habits, such as a proper diet, an exercise routine, and a positive attitude, people should enjoy better health. As research continues and cures are found for major health problems, life expectancy will be even longer. Aging is a normal process, beginning at infancy and continuing throughout the life cycle. As one grows older more health problems are likely to occur.

Changes experienced by the elderly

Biological and physiological changes occur that conflict with the action of drugs. Drug interactions are twice as likely to occur in the older age-group than in middle to adult life. These biological and physiological changes also affect the metabolism and excretion of drugs. Chronic conditions, such as hypertension, diabetes, heart conditions, and arthritis, interfere with homeostasis and may cause drugs to be less effective. These changes in concert with a person's genetic programming add to the severity of the health problems. It is difficult for a person who has had an active, productive life to deal with these changes. The nurse must be understanding to assist a person to adapt to a limited life-style.

Physical illness affects the mental posture of a person, which adds to anxiety and further deterioration. It is not uncommon for a person to feel unable to make the most basic decisions. The nurse, in collaboration with other members of the health team, can assist the patient, the family, and the person(s) responsible for giving care to understand the process of change.

Problems of the elderly

Some older persons are in the habit of visiting an internist for an annual physical examination. Since the elderly have more aches and pains than other age-groups, they may also visit a physician in family practice to deal with minor problems as they occur. If these aches and pains do not disappear, they may visit a third physician. Providing each physician writes a prescription(s), the patient may end up with several medications that duplicate their actions or that cause drug interaction or overdosage.

The patient should be encouraged to visit only one physician unless referred to a specialist. Should the patient visit another physician, he or she should prepare a list of all medications taken routinely or as needed and give it to the new physician. The physician can then prescribe medication and instruct the patient to delete duplicated medications or cause drug interactions.

Many older people live in poverty or have a very limited income. In order to lower medical costs they may reduce the amount of a prescription drug so that it will last longer. They may also stop taking the medication if they perceive it to be ineffective. They may go to the drug store and buy nonprescription drugs. Such drugs will save a physician's fee and are less expensive than prescription drugs, but they may be ineffective. However, the patient may perceive them to be a cure. Another method used to lower costs of drugs is to use a medication of a family member or friend. Misuse of drugs is widespread among the elderly and may cause various problems, such as fluid imbalance, nutritional disturbances, or psychological and neurological problems.

As older persons become forgetful, they may not take their medications or may not take them at the prescribed time. Often family members find medications on the floor, and they do not know whether the medication was taken or not.

When it becomes unsafe for the elderly person to stay at home alone, a day care center can relieve the pressure of family members who are employed. People enjoy being with others of their age to discuss memories and similar experiences. They can join in crafts and activities as they wish. There are opportunities to discuss thoughts and concerns with personnel at the center. The medication regime can be continued during the day, meals are served, and activities are planned. The activities at the center stimulate the elderly and give them something interesting to discuss at home in the evening.

More of the elderly are electing to live in their own home rather than in a retirement home or a nursing home. Sometimes they share their home with someone near their age. If an elderly person or a couple cannot care for themselves, they may choose to share their home with an individual or a couple who will not only be homemakers but give care as needed. Apart from providing a home for the one(s) giving care, a monetary compensation may be provided.

Medical alert system

A medical alert system is a valuable tool for the homebound person living alone or if the caregiver must be away for a few minutes. It is also used in retirement homes. In an emergency a button is pushed on the monitoring system or on a chain worn by the patient. The system alerts medical personnel to an emergency situation. Such a system gives a feeling of security to homebound persons and their families.

Medications for the elderly in the home

When purchasing medications from the pharmacy, elderly persons should request that childproof containers *not* be used. Containers that are available to prepare medications for a day or a week at a time should be purchased and used. The sections provide a special compartment for each hour the medications are to be given. The time can be written on the lid of the individual compartment and is easily removed if the time changes. These containers are especially helpful if someone outside the home assists the patient in preparing medications. These sectioned containers can be labeled as to the time the medication is to be taken.

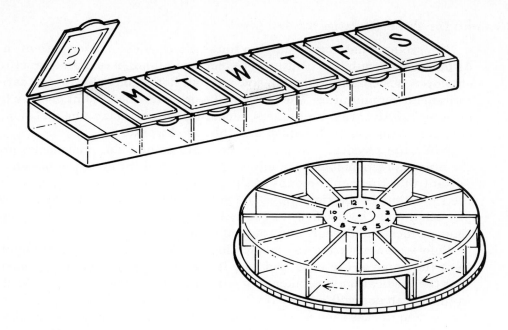

An appointment book with the day and date, a spiral notebook, or a tablet with the day and date added can be an efficient and safe way to plan medications taken in the home. The medications and the times they are to be taken each day are listed. The entry is crossed off after the medication has been taken.

Thursday, January 17, 1991
Motrin 300 mg after each meal
  8:00 AM 1:00 PM 6:00 PM
Naprosyn 250 mg two times a day
  8:00 AM 4:00 PM
Persantin 25 mg two times a day
  10:00 AM 6:00 PM
Lanoxin 40 mg daily
  10:00 AM
Mylanta 2 tablespoons after meals

The used medication sheet is discarded and a new one completed each day.

The visiting nurse

At such time that the patient, the family, or the person giving care feels that an assessment of the patient's health status is needed, a request can be made to the physician for assistance from a visiting nurse. The visiting nurse provides skilled care and consultation in the home under the supervision of the patient's physician.

The nurse assesses the patient's condition, gives nursing care as needed, and assists the family and the person giving care to better understand the patient. The nurse should review the patient's medication regimen with the person giving care. If some time has elapsed since the medication was ordered, the nurse should review the medication orders with the physician. The service provided by the visiting nurse will help the patient and family to feel secure that the patient is receiving optimum health care in the home. For the patient 65 years or older, the fees for the service usually will be paid by Medicare.

Medication for the elderly in the hospital

The professional nurse will plan nursing care for the older patient in the hospital. As our older population continues to increase in numbers, nurse practitioners will be employed not only in hospitals and nursing homes but also in day care centers and retirement communities. The nurse will work with the patient and the family, as well as other health care practitioners, including the physician, the dietitian, the pharmacist, the occupational therapist, and the social worker.

While the physician orders the medications and the pharmacist prepares them, the nurse is responsible for administering the medication to the patient. It is very important that the right amount of the right medicine be given to the right patient at the right time in the right way. The patient must also be observed for reactions. The physician must be notified if drug reactions occur. The nurse must record the date, time, medication, dosage, and route of administration.

Before administering the medication to the patient, the nurse should tell the patient the name of the drug and why it was prescribed. The nurse must also be sure that the medication was taken. Sometimes an older patient may hold the medication in the mouth and will remove it after the nurse leaves the bedside. They may save the medication in case they need it later. This could cause an overdose. The nurse should observe the patient after the administration of the medication for any unusual symptoms and record these observations on the patient's chart. The patient's physician must be notified if serious symptoms occur.

Administration of medications is one of the most important responsibilities of the nurse. However, without good skin care, oral hygiene, body alignment and exercise, and a well-balanced diet the patient will not maintain the potential for health and a satisfying life. Care of the whole person is essential for health and well-being.

Appendix

GLOSSARY

addends   the numbers to be added

ampule   a sealed glass container; usually contains one dose of the drug

capsule   a small soluble container for enclosing a single dose of medicine

complex fraction   a fraction whose numerator, denominator, or both contain fractions

decimal fraction   a fraction consisting of a numerator that is expressed in numericals, a decimal point that designates the value of the denominator, and the denominator, which is understood to be 10 or some power of 10

denominator   the number of parts into which a whole has been divided

difference   the result of subtracting

dividend   the number being divided

divisor   the number by which another number is divided

dosage   the determination and regulation of the size, frequency, and number of doses

dose   the exact amount of medicine to be administered at one time

drug   a chemical substance used in therapy, diagnosis, and prevention of a disease or condition

elixir   a clear, sweet, hydroalcoholic liquid in which a drug is suspended

equivalent   equal

fraction   indicates the number of equal parts of a whole

improper fraction   a fraction whose numerator is larger than or equal to the denominator

infusion   the therapeutic introduction of a fluid into a vein by the flow of gravity

injection   the therapeutic introduction of a fluid into a part of the body by force

integer   a whole number

intramuscular   within the muscle

intravenous   within the vein

invert   turn upside down

lowest common denominator   the smallest whole number that can be divided evenly by all denominators within the problem

medicine   any drug

milliequivalent   the number of grams of a solute contained in one milliliter of a normal solution

minuend   the number from which another number is subtracted

mixed number   a combination of a whole number and a proper fraction

multiplicand   the number that is to be multiplied

multiplier   the number that another number is to be multiplied by

numerator   the number of parts of a divided whole

oral dosage   a medication taken by mouth

parenteral dosage   a dosage administered by routes that bypass the gastrointestinal tract and that are generally given by injection

percent   indicates the number of hundredths

product   the result of multiplying

proper fraction   a fraction whose numerator is smaller than the denominator

proportion   two ratios that are of equal value and are connected by a double colon

quotient   the answer to a division problem

ratio   the relationship between two numbers that are connected by a colon

reconstitution   the return of a medication to its previous state by the addition of water

subcutaneous   beneath the skin

subtrahend   the number being subtracted

sum   the result of adding

suspension   a liquid in which a drug is distributed

syrup   a sweet, thick, aqueous liquid in which a drug is suspended

tablet   a drug compressed into a small disk

unit   the amount of a drug needed to produce a given result

vial   a glass container with a rubber stopper; usually contains a number of doses of a drug

ABBREVIATIONS AND SYMBOLS

$\overline{aa}$	of each	L	liter
a.c.	before meals	lb	pound
A.M.	morning, before noon	liq.	liquid
aq.	water	♏, m	minim
A.S.A.	acetylsalicylic acid (aspirin)	mcg, μg	microgram
b.i.d.	twice a day	mEq	milliequivalent
C	Celsius, centigrade	mg	milligram
$\overline{c}$	with	Mg	magnesium
Ca	calcium	min	minute
$CaCl_2$	calcium chloride	ml	milliliter
cap(s)	capsule	Na	sodium
cc	cubic centimeter	NaCl	sodium chloride
Cl	chlorine	$NaHCO_3$	sodium bicarbonate
d/c	discontinue	NPO	nothing by mouth
dil.	dilute	N.S.	normal saline
D.W.	dextrose water; distilled water	OD	right eye
		OS	left eye
elix.	elixir	OU	both eyes
F	Fahrenheit	oz	ounce
$FeSO_4$	ferrous sulfate	p.c.	after meals
fl.	fluid	per	by
gal	gallon	P.M.	after noon
Gm, gm	gram	p.o.	orally
gr	grain	p.r.n.	as needed
gtt	drops	pt	pint
h.	hour	q.	every
H_2O	water	q.d.	once a day
H_2O_2	hydrogen peroxide	q.h.	every hour
h.s.	at bedtime	q.i.d.	four times a day
I	iodine	q.o.d.	every other day
I.M.	intramuscular	q.o.h.	every other hour
inf.	infusion	qt	quart
inj.	injection	℞	a medical prescription
I.V.	intravenous	$\overline{s}$	without
I.V.P.B.	intravenous piggy back	sc	subcutaneous
I.V.S.S.	intravenous soluset	sol.	solution
K	potassium	S.O.S.	once if necessary
KCl	potassium chloride	SQ	subcutaneous
kg	kilogram	ss	on half

STAT, stat	immediately	tsp.	teaspoon
subq.	subcutaneous	U	unit
susp.	suspension	µg, mcg	microgram
syr.	syrup	ʒ	dram
tab	tablet	ʒ	ounce
Tbsp.	tablespoon	>	greater than
t.i.d.	three times a day	<	less than
tr., tinct.	tincture	/	per

CELSIUS AND FAHRENHEIT

EQUIVALENTS

Celsius (C)	Fahrenheit (F)
34.0	93.2
34.2	93.5
34.4	93.9
34.6	94.2
34.8	94.6
35.0	95.0
35.2	95.3
35.4	95.7
35.6	96.0
35.8	96.4
36.0	96.8
36.2	97.1
36.4	97.5
36.6	97.8
36.8	98.2
37.0	98.6
37.2	98.9
37.4	99.3
37.6	99.6
37.8	100.0
38.0	100.4
38.2	100.7
38.4	101.1
38.6	101.4
38.8	101.8
39.0	102.2
39.2	102.5
39.4	102.9
39.6	103.2
39.8	103.6
40.0	104.0
40.2	104.3
40.4	104.7
40.6	105.0
40.8	105.4
41.0	105.8
41.2	106.1
41.4	106.5
41.6	106.8
41.8	107.2
42.0	107.6
42.2	107.9

CONVERSION

FAHRENHEIT TO CENTIGRADE

$$C = \text{unknown}$$
change 98.6° F to centrigrade
$$C:F - 32::5:9$$
$$C:98.6 - 32::5:9$$
$$C:66.6 = 5:9$$
$$9C = 333$$
$$C = 37° \ C$$

or:

$$\text{Temperature} - 32 \times \frac{5}{9}$$

$$98.6 - 32 \times \frac{5}{9}$$

$$66.6 \times \frac{5}{9} = 37° \ C$$

CENTIGRADE TO FAHRENHEIT

$$F = \text{unknown}$$
Change 37° C to Fahrenheit
$$C:F - 32::5:9$$
$$37:F - 32::5:9$$
$$5F = 333 + 5 \times 32$$
$$5F = 333 + 160$$
$$F = 98.6° \ F$$

or:

$$\frac{9}{5} \times \text{Temperature} + 32$$

$$\frac{9}{5} \times 37 + 32$$

$$66.6 + 32 = 98.6° \ F$$

MATHEMATICS PRETEST

Define and give one example of each of the following:

1. Improper fraction_____

_____

Example:_____

2. Complex fraction_____

_____

Example:_____

3. Ratio_____

_____

Example:_____

4. Divisor_____

_____

Example:_____

5. Decimal fraction_____

_____

Example:_____

Add and reduce fractions to lowest terms.

6. $\frac{3}{8} + \frac{1}{3} =$

7. $2\frac{3}{7} + 1\frac{2}{3}$

8. $\frac{4}{5} + \frac{5}{9} =$

9. $1\frac{3}{5} + \frac{7}{8}/\frac{1}{3} =$

Add.

10. $1.03 + 2.2 + 1.134 =$

11. $30.962 + 0.57 + 2.3 =$

12. $6.88 + 4.5 + 1.678 =$

13. $1.479 + 28.68 + 4.5 =$

Subtract and reduce fractions to lowest terms.

14. $2\frac{1}{4} - \frac{7}{9}/\frac{2}{3} =$

15. $\frac{14}{15} - \frac{1}{6} =$

16. $5\frac{1}{4} - 4\frac{5}{8} =$

17. $2\frac{1}{3} - \frac{1}{2} =$

Subtract.

18. $2.04 - 0.987 =$

19. $43.597 - 42.843 =$

20. $8.53 - 7.945 =$

21. $2.006 - 0.589 =$

Multiply and reduce fractions to lowest terms.

22. $3 \times \frac{4}{7} =$

23. $\frac{2}{3} \times \frac{5}{6} =$

24. $2\frac{1}{2} \times 3\frac{3}{5} =$

25. $4\frac{7}{10} \times 1\frac{3}{4} =$

Multiply.

26. $3.47 \times 7.9 =$

27. $0.315 \times 5.8 =$

28. $4.884 \times 6.51 =$

29. $235 \times 6.72 =$

Divide and reduce fractions to lowest terms.

30. $\frac{3}{5} \div \frac{5}{6} =$

31. $\frac{1}{8} \div \frac{3}{10} =$

32. $\frac{1}{150} \div \frac{1}{20} =$

33. $2\frac{3}{4} \div 6\frac{2}{3} =$

Divide.

34. 241.73 ÷ 9.3 =

35. 0.9412 ÷ 4.16 =

36. 128.24 ÷ 6 =

37. 22.67 ÷ 3.5 =

Encircle the decimal fraction that has the *least* value.

38. 0.3, 0.03, 0.003

39. 0.1, 0.15, 0.155

40. 0.9, 0.45, 0.66

41. 0.4, 0.8, 0.21

42. 0.72, 0.721, 0.0072

Change the following fractions to decimals.

43. ⅝

44. ¾

45. ¹¹⁄₂₀

46. ¹⁷⁄₂₅

Change the following decimals to fractions reduced to lowest terms.

47. 0.875

48. 0.375

49. 0.05

50. 0.125

Calculate the following problems.

51. Express 0.432 as a percent.

52. Express 65% as a proper fraction and reduce to the lowest terms.

53. Express 0.3% as a ratio.

54. Express ⅛ as a percent.

55. What percent of 2.5 is 0.5?

56. What percent of ¾ is ⅜?

57. What percent of 160 is 12?

58. What is ¼% of 60?

59. What is 4½% of 940?

60. What is 65% of 450?

Change the following fractions and decimals to ratios reduced to lowest terms.

61. $^9\!/_{42}$　　　　　　　**62.** $1\frac{1}{2}/2\frac{2}{3}$　　　　　　　**63.** 0.8225

64. $^{125}\!/_{275}$　　　　　　　**65.** 0.34

Find the value of x.

66. $7:\!^7\!/_{100}::x:4$　　　　　**67.** $x:40::7:56$　　　　　**68.** $2.5:6::10:x$

69. $x:\frac{1}{4}\%::9.6:\frac{1}{300}$　　　**70.** $\frac{1}{150}:\frac{1}{100}::x:30$　　　**71.** $25:x::5:400$

72. $0.10:0.20::x:200$　　**73.** $\frac{1}{200}:\frac{1}{40}::100:x$　　**74.** $x:85::6:10$

75. $\frac{1}{20}/\frac{1}{5}:5::x:50$

ANSWERS

FRACTIONS—PRETEST, pp. 3-5

1. $^{19}\!/_{24}$
2. $1^{10}\!/_{63}$
3. $9^{7}\!/_{20}$
4. $10^{2}\!/_{3}$
5. $9^{3}\!/_{4}$
6. $5^{9}\!/_{16}$
7. $9^{1}\!/_{22}$
8. $7^{8}\!/_{9}$
9. $3^{5}\!/_{6}$
10. $5^{23}\!/_{24}$

11. $^{3}\!/_{10}$
12. $^{7}\!/_{8}$
13. $^{13}\!/_{15}$
14. $2^{5}\!/_{8}$
15. $6^{3}\!/_{26}$
16. $2^{17}\!/_{24}$
17. $1^{5}\!/_{6}$
18. $1^{4}\!/_{5}$
19. $1^{5}\!/_{16}$
20. $1^{5}\!/_{6}$

21. $^{1}\!/_{15}$
22. $^{21}\!/_{80}$
23. 5
24. $7^{19}\!/_{63}$
25. $1^{1}\!/_{14}$
26. $^{1}\!/_{10,000}$
27. $4^{5}\!/_{18}$
28. $5^{41}\!/_{75}$
29. $12^{1}\!/_{12}$
30. $2^{25}\!/_{28}$

31. $^{5}\!/_{16}$
32. $^{49}\!/_{81}$
33. $1^{1}\!/_{3}$
34. $33^{1}\!/_{3}$
35. $^{7}\!/_{8}$
36. $1^{1}\!/_{3}$
37. $^{1}\!/_{12}$
38. $^{5}\!/_{9}$
39. $1^{7}\!/_{10}$
40. 2

FRACTIONS—WORK SHEET, pp. 17-24

Improper fractions to mixed numbers, pp. 17-18

1. $1^{1}\!/_{3}$
2. 3
3. $2^{1}\!/_{4}$
4. $3^{1}\!/_{5}$
5. $1^{7}\!/_{10}$
6. $1^{1}\!/_{2}$

7. $1^{3}\!/_{7}$
8. $3^{1}\!/_{4}$
9. $3^{1}\!/_{3}$
10. $2^{1}\!/_{9}$
11. $1^{1}\!/_{2}$
12. $1^{1}\!/_{8}$

13. $1^{2}\!/_{3}$
14. $2^{1}\!/_{6}$
15. $6^{1}\!/_{3}$
16. $3^{1}\!/_{7}$
17. $2^{9}\!/_{13}$
18. $3^{1}\!/_{2}$

19. $4^{2}\!/_{3}$
20. $1^{3}\!/_{8}$
21. $3^{1}\!/_{2}$
22. $1^{3}\!/_{25}$
23. $2^{7}\!/_{15}$
24. $1^{1}\!/_{2}$

Mixed numbers to improper fractions, pp. 18-19

1. $^{3}\!/_{2}$
2. $^{15}\!/_{4}$
3. $^{8}\!/_{3}$
4. $^{33}\!/_{8}$
5. $^{65}\!/_{9}$
6. $^{53}\!/_{10}$

7. $^{17}\!/_{6}$
8. $^{8}\!/_{5}$
9. $^{25}\!/_{7}$
10. $^{22}\!/_{3}$
11. $^{39}\!/_{8}$
12. $^{11}\!/_{2}$

13. $^{29}\!/_{3}$
14. $^{70}\!/_{11}$
15. $^{307}\!/_{100}$
16. $^{31}\!/_{7}$
17. $^{4}\!/_{3}$
18. $^{27}\!/_{10}$

19. $^{53}\!/_{8}$
20. $^{29}\!/_{13}$
21. $^{28}\!/_{25}$
22. $^{17}\!/_{4}$
23. $^{43}\!/_{8}$
24. $^{22}\!/_{9}$

Addition, pp. 19-20

1. $1^{1}\!/_{2}$
2. $^{29}\!/_{35}$
3. $3^{19}\!/_{24}$
4. $1^{8}\!/_{9}$
5. $3^{1}\!/_{4}$
6. $^{65}\!/_{77}$

7. $5^{13}\!/_{20}$
8. $3^{5}\!/_{39}$
9. $3^{7}\!/_{16}$
10. $10^{4}\!/_{5}$
11. $6^{1}\!/_{2}$
12. $6^{14}\!/_{15}$

13. $7^{5}\!/_{8}$
14. $6^{17}\!/_{22}$
15. $6^{4}\!/_{9}$
16. $6^{11}\!/_{30}$
17. $4^{17}\!/_{24}$
18. $6^{19}\!/_{40}$

19. $6^{19}\!/_{30}$
20. $1^{7}\!/_{12}$
21. $4^{3}\!/_{20}$
22. 9
23. $6^{10}\!/_{63}$
24. $8^{7}\!/_{30}$

Subtraction, pp. 20-21

1. $^{5}\!/_{21}$
2. $^{9}\!/_{16}$
3. $^{7}\!/_{48}$
4. $^{1}\!/_{2}$
5. $^{1}\!/_{5}$
6. $^{3}\!/_{16}$

7. $1^{1}\!/_{10}$
8. $1^{1}\!/_{6}$
9. $2^{31}\!/_{40}$
10. $1^{1}\!/_{24}$
11. $^{11}\!/_{16}$
12. $1^{13}\!/_{24}$

13. $1^{15}\!/_{16}$
14. $^{5}\!/_{8}$
15. $1^{1}\!/_{3}$
16. $2^{5}\!/_{8}$
17. $^{19}\!/_{24}$
18. $1^{25}\!/_{48}$

19. $1^{5}\!/_{12}$
20. $1^{7}\!/_{24}$
21. $1^{1}\!/_{12}$
22. $1^{19}\!/_{24}$
23. $1^{3}\!/_{5}$
24. $^{15}\!/_{16}$

Multiplication, pp. 21-23

1. $^{4}\!/_{15}$
2. $^{5}\!/_{27}$
3. $^{7}\!/_{12}$
4. $^{4}\!/_{7}$
5. 4
6. $1^{1}\!/_{2}$

7. $8^{3}\!/_{4}$
8. $6^{6}\!/_{35}$
9. $11^{7}\!/_{8}$
10. $5^{49}\!/_{50}$
11. $5^{2}\!/_{15}$
12. $12^{11}\!/_{16}$

13. $4^{4}\!/_{15}$
14. $1^{25}\!/_{32}$
15. $5^{5}\!/_{8}$
16. $^{1}\!/_{5}$
17. $4^{15}\!/_{32}$
18. $^{3}\!/_{1000}$

19. $4^{1}\!/_{10}$
20. $4^{1}\!/_{4}$
21. $2^{11}\!/_{14}$
22. $6^{5}\!/_{12}$
23. $3^{2}\!/_{3}$
24. $3^{1}\!/_{9}$

Division, pp. 23-24

1. $^{10}/_{21}$	**7.** $2\frac{1}{2}$	**13.** $1^{29}/_{40}$	**19.** $1^{13}/_{22}$
2. $1\frac{4}{5}$	**8.** $1^{23}/_{26}$	**14.** $3^{47}/_{51}$	**20.** $2^{1}/_{16}$
3. $2\frac{1}{5}$	**9.** $2^{32}/_{39}$	**15.** $1^{29}/_{176}$	**21.** $2^{2}/_{19}$
4. $2\frac{5}{6}$	**10.** $1^{7}/_{20}$	**16.** $3\frac{1}{2}$	**22.** $1^{9}/_{28}$
5. $1\frac{5}{9}$	**11.** $1^{7}/_{11}$	**17.** $2^{5}/_{17}$	**23.** $1\frac{1}{2}$
6. $2^{23}/_{56}$	**12.** $1\frac{7}{8}$	**18.** $4^{23}/_{24}$	**24.** $1^{22}/_{23}$

FRACTIONS—POSTTEST 1, pp. 25-27

1. $1\frac{1}{9}$	**11.** $^{5}/_{36}$	**21.** $^{9}/_{14}$	**31.** $1^{1}/_{15}$
2. $^{17}/_{24}$	**12.** $^{9}/_{10}$	**22.** $2\frac{2}{5}$	**32.** 10
3. $5^{1}/_{12}$	**13.** $^{5}/_{6}$	**23.** $^{2}/_{5}$	**33.** $^{2}/_{3}$
4. $4^{3}/_{10}$	**14.** $^{3}/_{14}$	**24.** 2	**34.** $1\frac{1}{4}$
5. $3^{2}/_{21}$	**15.** $1\frac{1}{9}$	**25.** $3^{5}/_{24}$	**35.** $^{3}/_{20}$
6. $4^{10}/_{21}$	**16.** $1^{15}/_{16}$	**26.** $3\frac{1}{3}$	**36.** $^{9}/_{14}$
7. $^{39}/_{50}$	**17.** $1^{31}/_{63}$	**27.** $14^{7}/_{10}$	**37.** $^{3}/_{5}$
8. $3^{19}/_{24}$	**18.** $1^{9}/_{20}$	**28.** $3^{18}/_{35}$	**38.** $1^{7}/_{20}$
9. $8^{3}/_{20}$	**19.** $5^{7}/_{10}$	**29.** $^{7}/_{8}$	**39.** $4\frac{1}{2}$
10. $7^{7}/_{12}$	**20.** $1^{1}/_{12}$	**30.** $42\frac{1}{2}$	**40.** $1^{3}/_{22}$

FRACTIONS—POSTTEST 2, pp. 29-31

1. $1^{1}/_{12}$	**11.** $^{1}/_{9}$	**21.** $^{4}/_{21}$	**31.** $^{27}/_{32}$
2. $4^{1}/_{10}$	**12.** $1\frac{7}{8}$	**22.** $6\frac{1}{5}$	**32.** $^{21}/_{26}$
3. $3^{2}/_{21}$	**13.** $1^{5}/_{6}$	**23.** $1\frac{1}{3}$	**33.** $6^{2}/_{9}$
4. $7^{1}/_{15}$	**14.** $^{32}/_{35}$	**24.** $7^{21}/_{22}$	**34.** $^{1}/_{49}$
5. $5^{11}/_{40}$	**15.** $2^{5}/_{16}$	**25.** $1^{17}/_{18}$	**35.** $^{5}/_{8}$
6. $4^{19}/_{24}$	**16.** $^{5}/_{8}$	**26.** $^{1}/_{1000}$	**36.** $^{21}/_{32}$
7. $11\frac{1}{5}$	**17.** $1\frac{1}{2}$	**27.** $6^{6}/_{11}$	**37.** $1^{23}/_{32}$
8. $6^{25}/_{36}$	**18.** $3^{9}/_{10}$	**28.** 36	**38.** $1^{11}/_{16}$
9. $3\frac{1}{2}$	**19.** $^{3}/_{5}$	**29.** $3\frac{1}{2}$	**39.** $1^{19}/_{26}$
10. $3^{19}/_{40}$	**20.** $4^{13}/_{14}$	**30.** $11\frac{1}{4}$	**40.** $1\frac{1}{8}$

DECIMALS—PRETEST, pp. 33-36

1. Four hundredths
2. One and six tenths
3. Sixteen and six thousand seven hundred thirty-four hundred thousandths
4. One and fifteen thousandths
5. Nine thousandths

6. 0.02	**23.** 1.008	**39.** 0.676	**55.** $^{161}/_{500}$
7. 0.004	**24.** 759.4	**40.** 356.546	**56.** $^{27}/_{100}$
8. 1.6	**25.** 1.7	**41.** 0.21	**57.** $^{3}/_{10}$
9. 2.082	**26.** 11.69	**42.** 17.95	**58.** $^{1}/_{250}$
10. 0.003	**27.** 0.079	**43.** 3.94	**59.** $^{17}/_{50}$
11. 1429.421	**28.** 10.946	**44.** 31,000	**60.** $^{19}/_{20}$
12. 983.799	**29.** 0.48	**45.** 0.01	**61.** 0.6
13. 25.376	**30.** 8.06	**46.** 8.98	**62.** 0.67
14. 324.3	**31.** 0.0567	**47.** 627	**63.** 0.01
15. 36.1094	**32.** 6.6472	**48.** 0.70	**64.** 0.35
16. 1012.867	**33.** 0.0608	**49.** 40.75	**65.** 0.08
17. 150.6736	**34.** 0.193272	**50.** 0.02	**66.** 0.625, 0.63
18. 1003.6135	**35.** 1.9425	**51.** $^{1}/_{5}$	**67.** 0.03
19. 84.565	**36.** 3.2604	**52.** $^{9}/_{20}$	**68.** 0.375, 0.38
20. 552.1326	**37.** 29.5336	**53.** $^{1}/_{125}$	**69.** 0.01
21. 1.078	**38.** 186.543	**54.** $^{1}/_{4}$	**70.** 0.16
22. 863.45			

DECIMALS—WORK SHEET, pp. 43-44

1. Two tenths
2. Nine and sixty-eight hundredths
3. One hundred eighty-six and nine hundred thirty-five thousandths
4. Eight one hundred thousandths
5. Eighty-six thousand nine hundred thirty-one hundred thousandths
6. Six hundred ninety-eight thousand four hundred thirty-seven and fifteen hundredths
7. Three ten thousandths
8. Twelve thousand three hundred seventy-five and seven tenths
9. Six and four thousandths

10. One thousand nine hundred sixty-eight and three hundred forty-two thousandths
11. Two hundredths
12. Thirty-five and four thousand seven hundred twenty-six ten thousandths

13. 0.25	**16.** 0.68	**19.** 0.6	**22.** 0.08
14. 0.45	**17.** 1.8	**20.** 0.0003	**23.** 0.007
15. 0.98	**18.** 7.44	**21.** 1.0022	**24.** 3.006

Addition, pp. 44-45

1. 41.755	**7.** 21.919	**13.** 22.833	**19.** 526.173
2. 372.675	**8.** 16.908	**14.** 111.5919	**20.** 55.117
3. 40.9787	**9.** 54.033	**15.** 26.62	**21.** 216.28
4. 888.5997	**10.** 894.842	**16.** 23.391	**22.** 51.555
5. 39.073	**11.** 67.137	**17.** 41.4281	**23.** 142.218
6. 27.851	**12.** 37.394	**18.** 37.9	**24.** 218.05

Subtraction, pp. 45-46

1. 1257.87	**7.** 1.079	**13.** 50.675	**19.** 0.88
2. 1.849	**8.** 4.144	**14.** 62.022	**20.** 0.009
3. 0.71	**9.** 0.461	**15.** 287.371	**21.** 919.57
4. 32.746	**10.** 0.988	**16.** 0.187	**22.** 659.74
5. 174.804	**11.** 3.332	**17.** 9.949	**23.** 0.447
6. 7.418	**12.** 6.893	**18.** 2.939	**24.** 17.67

Multiplication, pp. 46-47

1. 115.3674	**9.** 56.1144	**17.** 13,282.75
2. 16.25	**10.** 41.92	**18.** 409.0318
3. 159.84	**11.** 11.696	**19.** 0.512
4. 6.56	**12.** 1.156	**20.** 43.472
5. 609.6	**13.** 33.6813	**21.** 643211.7
6. 52.052	**14.** 35.7	**22.** 0.15113
7. 26.25	**15.** 33.6	**23.** 7147.5
8. 696	**16.** 103.983	**24.** 23.5971

Multiply by 10, p. 48

1. 0.9	**4.** 3.0		
2. 2.0	**5.** 6.25		
3. 1.8	**6.** 23.3		

Multiply by 100, p. 48

1. 2.3	**4.** 12.5
2. 150	**5.** 865
3. 0.4	**6.** 7640

Multiply by 1000, p. 48

1. 200	**4.** 9650
2. 5	**5.** 460
3. 187	**6.** 489

Multiply by 0.1, p. 48

1. 3.0	**4.** 0.095
2. 0.069	**5.** 0.0138
3. 0.17	**6.** 0.567

Multiply by 0.01, p. 48

1. 0.0026	**4.** 0.112
2. 0.908	**5.** 0.00875
3. 0.055	**6.** 0.633

Multiply by 0.001, p. 48

1. 0.056	**4.** 0.0333
2. 0.01255	**5.** 0.009684
3. 0.1265	**6.** 0.241

Round to the nearest tenth, p. 48

1. 0.3	**4.** 0.7
2. 0.9	**5.** 58.4
3. 2.4	**6.** 8.1

Round to the nearest hundredth, p. 48

1. 2.56	**4.** 3.92
2. 4.28	**5.** 6.53
3. 0.28	**6.** 2.99

Round to the nearest thousandth, p. 48

1. 27.863	**4.** 0.849
2. 5.925	**5.** 321.087
3. 2.157	**6.** 455.768

Division, pp. 48-50

1. 1.17	**7.** 1.7	**13.** 740	**19.** 0.48
2. 4140	**8.** 0.13	**14.** 0.05	**20.** 0.8
3. 7.8	**9.** 185	**15.** 0.5	**21.** 2.52
4. 0.03	**10.** 0.02	**16.** 4.53	**22.** 2.63
5. 400	**11.** 0.13	**17.** 1.45	**23.** 47
6. 8.4	**12.** 82.6	**18.** 17.39	**24.** 17.48

Divide by 10, p. 50

1. 0.6	**4.** 0.005
2. 0.02	**5.** 0.0375
3. 0.98	**6.** 0.099

Divide by 100, p. 50

1. 0.007	**4.** 0.0019
2. 0.0811	**5.** 0.12
3. 7	**6.** 0.302

Divide by 1000, p. 50

1. 0.0018	**4.** 0.0546
2. 0.36	**5.** 0.0075
3. 0.00025	**6.** 7.14

Divide by 0.1, p. 50

1. 28	**4.** 9.87
2. 1	**5.** 150
3. 6.5	**6.** 82.5

Divide by 0.01, p. 50

1. 3600	**4.** 959
2. 16	**5.** 80
3. 48	**6.** 9.7

Divide by 0.001, p. 50

1. 6200	**4.** 860
2. 839,000	**5.** 13,800
3. 5000	**6.** 15.6

Decimal fractions to proper fractions, pp. 50-51

1. ³⁄₅₀
2. ¹⁹⁄₂₀₀
3. ⁴⁄₅
4. ¹⁷⁄₂₅
5. ⅛
6. ³⁷⁄₅₀

7. ¹⁄₄₀₀
8. ¹⁷⁄₂₀
9. ½
10. ⅝
11. ¼
12. ⁹⁄₁₀

13. ¹⁄₂₅₀
14. ³⁄₂₅
15. ¹¹⁄₂₀₀
16. ⅞
17. ¹⁶⁄₂₅
18. ¾

19. ⁴⁄₂₅
20. ¹¹⁄₅₀
21. ¹⁄₂₀₀
22. ¹⁄₁₀₀
23. ¹¹⁄₂₅₀
24. ⅕

Proper fractions to decimal fractions, pp. 51-52

1. 0.125, 0.13
2. 0.55
3. 0.67
4. 0.375, 0.38
5. 0.64
6. 0.25

7. 0.24
8. 0.6
9. 0.04
10. 0.33
11. 0.86
12. 0.08

13. 0.5
14. 0.9
15. 0.8
16. 0.15
17. 0.875, 0.88
18. 0.25

19. 0.75
20. 0.34
21. 0.01
22. 0.09
23. 0.83
24. 0.95

DECIMALS—POSTTEST 1, pp. 53-56

1. Forty-two and sixty-eight thousand five hundred nineth-three hundred thousandths
2. Six hundred thirty-four and eighteen hundredths
3. Nine tenths
4. Three thousandths
5. Sixty-four and two hundred thirty-one thousandths
6. 0.25
7. 0.15
8. 0.6666
9. 0.6
10. 5.5
11. 54.66
12. 8.235
13. 926.043
14. 22.904
15. 8.89
16. 2054.74
17. 138.44
18. 6.352
19. 6.104
20. 2152.626
21. 88.982
22. 7.137
23. 0.339
24. 5.32
25. 1.4532
26. 323.08
27. 0.628

28. 20.95
29. 43.6077
30. 0.211
31. 702.4472
32. 0.13904
33. 5.46875
34. 2366.079981
35. 162
36. 0.850304
37. 44.278
38. 0.585
39. 924448.47552
40. 21.892
41. 16.8
42. 4662.5
43. 1481.67
44. 1880
45. 51333.33
46. 627
47. 1.41
48. 55.19
49. 2

50. 500
51. ⁹⁄₁₀₀
52. ⅝
53. ⁴⁄₂₅
54. ½
55. ¹⁄₄₀₀
56. ¹¹⁄₂₀
57. ⅜
58. ⅖
59. ³⁄₅₀₀
60. ¾
61. 0.71
62. 0.22
63. 0.85
64. 0.01
65. 0.8
66. 0.31
67. 0.33
68. 0.004
69. 0.125, 0.13
70. 0.09

DECIMALS—POSTTEST 2, pp. 57-60

1. Five tenths
2. Eight and two thousand six hundred fifty-eight ten thousandths
3. Four and two ten thousandths
4. One hundred twenty-three and sixty-nine hundredths
5. Two and four hundred five thousandths
6. 0.8
7. 0.9
8. 0.86
9. 0.659
10. 1.222
11. 456.8191
12. 130.5837
13. 16.055
14. 33.209
15. 280.895
16. 285.591
17. 2011.306
18. 47.725
19. 507.629
20. 339
21. 612.969

22. 27.9
23. 0.587
24. 7.789
25. 2.766
26. 2.513
27. 81.79
28. 3.84
29. 1.085
30. 223.98
31. 28.57704
32. 167.04
33. 104,552
34. 247.975
35. 27.61018
36. 1.01574
37. 276.35148

38. 83.2
39. 2560
40. 161.975
41. 820
42. 1.11
43. 5
44. 0.48
45. 4.08
46. 15,500
47. 2
48. 12
49. 0.30
50. 2.47
51. ¹⁄₂₅
52. ¹⁄₂₀₀
53. ⁷⁄₂₀

54. ⅛
55. 9/10
56. 17/20
57. 3/1000
58. 4/5
59. 11/50

60. ⅗
61. 0.55
62. 0.17
63. 0.003
64. 0.875, 0.88
65. 0.4

66. 0.75
67. 0.007
68. 0.5
69. 0.008
70. 0.19

PERCENTS—PRETEST, pp. 61-63

Fractions to percents, p. 61

1. 1⅔%, 1.6666%
2. 71³/₇%, 71.4285%
3. 12½%, 12.5%

4. 30%
5. 133⅓%, 133.3333%

Decimals to percents, p. 61

6. 0.6%
7. 35%
8. 42.7%

9. 382.1%
10. 70%

Percents to fractions, p. 62

11. 1/200
12. ¾
13. 19/200

14. 31/125
15. 3/800

Percents to decimals, p. 62

16. 0.0116
17. 0.075
18. 0.133

19. 0.0088
20. 0.63

What percent of, pp. 62-63

21. 375%
22. 16⅔%, 16.6666%
23. 65%
24. ⅕%, 0.2%
25. 33⅓%, 33.333%

26. 12³²/₁₈₉%, 12.1693%
27. 43⁷/₂₆%, 43.2692%
28. 10%
29. 7¹/₇%, 7.1428%
30. 1²⁰⁹/₂₉₁%, 1.7182%

What is, p. 63

31. 1.8
32. 0.15
33. 2.565
34. 0.68
35. 3.08

36. 4.278
37. 0.05999
38. 19.36
39. 11.856
40. 15

PERCENTS—WORK SHEET, pp. 69-75

Fractions to percents, pp. 69-70

1. 75%
2. 50%
3. 37½%
4. 80%
5. 32%
6. 3/10%

7. 3½%
8. 66⅔%
9. 41⅔%
10. 23⅓%
11. 2¼%
12. 84⅜%

13. 15%
14. 70¹⁰/₁₇%
15. 22⁸/₁₁%
16. 6%
17. 68¾%
18. 21³/₇%

19. 38²/₂₁%
20. 83⅓%
21. ¾%
22. 13⅓%
23. 44⁴/₉%
24. 87½%

Decimals to percents, pp. 70-71

1. 40.2%
2. 3.67%
3. 431%
4. 16.3%
5. 622%
6. 98%

7. 32.76%
8. 30%
9. 133.97%
10. 14.5%
11. 28.24%
12. 67%

13. 70%
14. 62.24%
15. 42%
16. 63.37%
17. 620%
18. 15.9%

19. 290.14%
20. 67.3%
21. 40.5%
22. 37.12%
23. 723.4%
24. 220%

Percents to fractions, pp. 71-72

1. 7/200
2. 3/400
3. 203/500
4. 1/800
5. 1/10
6. 1/150

7. 1/600
8. 7/2000
9. 9/20
10. 101/500
11. 1/160
12. 9/200

13. 3/25
14. 1/400
15. 19/800
16. 29/50
17. 2/25
18. 1/16

19. 21/1000
20. 3/2000
21. 1/200
22. 81/250
23. ⅔
24. 9/500

Percents to decimals, pp. 72-73

1. 0.375
2. 0.03
3. 0.017
4. 0.0675
5. 0.0042
6. 0.0025

7. 0.4
8. 0.0135
9. 0.025
10. 0.00375
11. 0.05
12. 0.8

13. 0.0023
14. 0.726
15. 0.16
16. 0.3064
17. 0.0293
18. 0.003125

19. 0.0875
20. 0.005
21. 0.0575
22. 0.0098
23. 0.069
24. 0.0058

What percent of, pp. 73-74

1. 55%
2. 16⅔%, 16.6666%
3. 7⅞%, 7.875%
4. 50%
5. 46⅔%, 46.6666%
6. 84%

7. 24⁶/₁₁%, 24.5454%
8. 200%
9. 5²⁵/₃₆%, 5.6944%
10. 2%
11. 12%
12. 5%

13. 15%
14. 23¹/₁₃%, 23.0769%
15. 74³⁸/₁₆₃%, 74.2331%
16. 20%
17. 10%
18. 4⁵⁶/₇₅%, 4.746%

19. 10¹⁵/₁₉%, 10.7894%
20. 45%
21. 1%
22. 2²/₂₅%, 2.08%
23. 3¾%, 3.75%
24. 20%

What is, pp. 74-75

1. 119.5
2. 3.4
3. 14.28
4. 633.75
5. 0.14
6. 1.625
7. 30.77
8. 999.9 or 1000
9. 1.995
10. 4.0
11. 11.52
12. 0.13
13. 0.585
14. 0.12
15. 131.712
16. 540.02
17. 0.17
18. 11.07
19. 168.48
20. 0.066
21. 10.752
22. 105
23. 0.10125
24. 5.0868

PERCENTS—POSTTEST 1, pp. 77-79

Fractions to percents, p. 77

1. $44\frac{4}{9}\%$, 44.4444%
2. $87\frac{1}{2}\%$, 87.5%
3. 55%
4. $266\frac{2}{3}\%$, 266.6666%
5. $\frac{3}{10}\%$, 0.3%

Decimals to percents, pp. 77

6. 25.6%
7. 3330%
8. 0.4%
9. 167.8%
10. 90%

Percents to fractions, p. 78

11. $\frac{3}{5}$
12. $\frac{17}{20}$
13. $\frac{3}{1000}$
14. $\frac{1}{400}$
15. $\frac{7}{200}$

Percents to decimals, p. 78

16. 0.863
17. 0.04625
18. 0.2945
19. 0.0875
20. 0.0036

What percent of, pp. 78-79

21. 10%
22. 5%
23. $\frac{1}{3}\%$, 0.33%
24. 12%
25. $42\frac{6}{7}\%$, 42.8571%
26. 20%
27. 50%
28. $7\frac{1}{2}\%$, 7.5%
29. $8\frac{6}{13}\%$, 8.4615%
30. 8%

What is, p. 79

31. 520
32. 36
33. 0.09
34. 170
35. 1.6875
36. 42.3
37. 292.5
38. 0.15
39. 2.408
40. 0.4576

PERCENTS—POSTTEST 2, pp. 81-83

Fractions to percents, p. 81

1. $12\frac{1}{2}\%$, 12.5%
2. 40%
3. $16\frac{2}{3}\%$, 16.6666%
4. 95%
5. $122\frac{2}{9}\%$, 122.2222%

Decimals to percents, p. 81

6. 6.5%
7. 0.5%
8. 434.6%
9. 57%
10. 20%

Percents to fractions, p. 82

11. $\frac{3}{1000}$
12. $\frac{33}{200}$
13. $\frac{3}{500}$
14. $\frac{7}{400}$
15. $\frac{1}{400}$

Percents to decimals, p. 82

16. 0.004
17. 0.0375
18. 0.07
19. 0.0555
20. 0.65

What percent of, pp. 82-83

21. $22\frac{2}{9}\%$, 22.2222%
22. 50%
23. $2\frac{2}{5}\%$, 2.4%
24. 80%
25. $7\frac{1}{2}\%$, 7.5%
26. 10%
27. $41\frac{7}{23}\%$, 41.3043%
28. $12\frac{1}{2}\%$, 12.5%
29. $40\frac{20}{87}\%$, 40.2298%
30. $126\frac{62}{63}\%$, 126.9841%

What is, p. 83

31. 227.5
32. 0.29
33. 42.3
34. 9.68
35. 14.4
36. 19.575
37. 10.9215
38. 0.56
39. 0.156
40. 97.232

RATIOS—PRETEST, p. 85

1. $\frac{1}{3}$, 0.3333, 33.33%
2. 143:200, $\frac{143}{200}$, 71.5%
3. 2:5, 0.4, 40%
4. 1:8, $\frac{1}{8}$, 0.125
5. $\frac{1}{20}$, 0.05, 5%
6. 5:32, 0.15625, 15.625%
7. 143:500, $\frac{143}{500}$, 28.6%
8. 5:7, $\frac{5}{7}$, 0.714
9. 13:80, $\frac{13}{80}$, 0.1625
10. 231:500, $\frac{231}{500}$, 46.2%

RATIOS—WORK SHEET, pp. 91-98

Fractions to ratios, pp. 91-92

1. 3:4
2. 1:3
3. 3:4
4. 2:3
5. 3:10
6. 1:2
7. 2:3
8. 14:25
9. 1:4
10. 2:5
11. 31:100
12. 1:2
13. 5:8
14. 3:2
15. 10:7
16. 1:4
17. 67:14
18. 16:27
19. 10:1
20. 7:30
21. 3:67
22. 155:228
23. 1:1
24. 25:112

Decimals to ratios, pp. 92-93

1. 112:125
2. 24:25
3. 3369:5000
4. 3:50
5. 189:250
6. 3:5
7. 252:625
8. 821:1000
9. 37:50
10. 83:500
11. 547:1250
12. 13:50
13. 123:250
14. 33:100
15. 41:50
16. 19:20
17. 1:5
18. 47:200
19. 67:100
20. 1071:2000
21. 423:500
22. 43:250
23. 9:10
24. 297:625

Percents to ratios, pp. 93-95

1. 1:10	**7.** 11:25	**13.** 1:40	**19.** 77:800
2. 1:40	**8.** 157:1000	**14.** 11:2500	**20.** 7:500
3. 1:3	**9.** 6:125	**15.** 1:2000	**21.** 3:500
4. 3:800	**10.** 2781:5000	**16.** 39:5000	**22.** 109:900
5. 1:4	**11.** 31:400	**17.** 1:100	**23.** 6:175
6. 27:1000	**12.** 7:20	**18.** 27:400	**24.** 41:500

Ratios to fractions, pp. 95-96

1. ½	**7.** $3/100$	**13.** $3\tfrac{1}{5}$	**19.** $1\tfrac{6}{11}$
2. ¾	**8.** 1½	**14.** ½	**20.** $37/67$
3. $1/16$	**9.** ⅓	**15.** ⅕	**21.** $3\tfrac{11}{63}$
4. ⅘	**10.** $1\tfrac{3}{7}$	**16.** $8/45$	**22.** $7/429$
5. $1/200$	**11.** 1	**17.** $26/51$	**23.** $82/127$
6. $1/50$	**12.** ⅓	**18.** ⅓	**24.** $121/821$

Ratios to decimal numbers, pp. 96-97

1. 0.5	**7.** 0.5	**13.** 0.5098	**19.** 0.3888
2. 0.25	**8.** 1.5	**14.** 0.9	**20.** 6240
3. 0.375	**9.** 0.0666	**15.** 0.2666	**21.** 2.9166
4. 0.625	**10.** 0.1	**16.** 0.5235	**22.** 12
5. 0.3333	**11.** 0.4	**17.** 0.027	**23.** 0.7777
6. 6.25	**12.** 0.4525	**18.** 0.4772	**24.** 3.5

Ratios to percent, pp. 97-99

1. 50%	**9.** $1/10$%, 0.1%	**17.** 95%
2. $3\tfrac{1}{33}$%, 3.0303%	**10.** 25%	**18.** $24\tfrac{8}{33}$%, 24.2424%
3. 10%	**11.** $56\tfrac{2}{3}$%, 56.6666%	**19.** $55\tfrac{5}{9}$%, 55.5555%
4. 20%	**12.** $206\tfrac{1}{4}$%, 206.25%	**20.** $31\tfrac{11}{19}$%, 31.5789%
5. $128\tfrac{4}{7}$%, 128.5714%	**13.** $52\tfrac{1}{12}$%, 52.0833%	**21.** 20%
6. $71\tfrac{3}{7}$%, 71.4285%	**14.** 225%	**22.** $2133\tfrac{1}{3}$%, 2133.3333%
7. $37\tfrac{1}{27}$%, 37.037%	**15.** ⅕%, 0.2%	**23.** $226\tfrac{2}{23}$%, 226.0869%
8. 175%	**16.** $66\tfrac{2}{3}$%, 66.6666%	**24.** $56\tfrac{12}{23}$%, 56.5217%

RATIOS—POSTTEST 1, p. 101

1. ⅞, 0.875, 87.5%	**5.** 7:20, $7/20$, 35%	**8.** 3:1000, $3/1000$, 0.003
2. 1:250, $1/250$, 0.4%	**6.** 6:25, 0.24, 24%	**9.** 41:200, $41/200$, 20.5%
3. 13:20, 0.65, 65%	**7.** $27/40$, 0.675, 67.5%	**10.** 4:11, 0.3636, 36.36%
4. 9:400, $9/400$, 0.0225		

RATIOS—POSTTEST 2, p. 103

1. $7/10$, 0.7, 70%	**5.** 3:800, $3/800$, 0.00375	**8.** $2/7$, 0.2857, 28.57%
2. 5:16, 0.3125, 31.25%	**6.** 1:150, 0.0066, 0.66%	**9.** 161:500, $161/500$, 32.2%
3. 3:40, $3/40$, 7.5%	**7.** 7:1000, $7/1000$, 0.7%	**10.** 91:500, $91/500$, 0.182
4. 3:50, $3/50$, 0.06		

PROPORTIONS—PRETEST, pp. 105-106

1. 100	**6.** 4	**11.** 80	**16.** 80
2. 7½ or 7.5	**7.** 400 or 399.9	**12.** ⅙	**17.** 10
3. $1/600$	**8.** ½	**13.** 14	**18.** 126
4. 3.2	**9.** $3/7$	**14.** 48	**19.** $1/150$
5. 128	**10.** 8	**15.** $3/10$	**20.** 16¼ or 16.25

PROPORTIONS—WORK SHEET, pp. 111-115

1. 84	**14.** 1½	**27.** ½ or 0.5
2. 600	**15.** 2000	**28.** 960
3. 28.125	**16.** 1	**29.** 25
4. 1⅕	**17.** 80	**30.** 20
5. 52½	**18.** 1	**31.** ½ or 0.5
6. 27	**19.** 2400	**32.** 1.2
7. 7200	**20.** 5	**33.** 1.17
8. 1½ or 1.5	**21.** 600	**34.** 3
9. ¾	**22.** 40	**35.** 15
10. 1	**23.** 0.032	**36.** 30
11. 4⅘	**24.** 128	**37.** 48
12. 252	**25.** 0.2	**38.** 15
13. 240	**26.** 8	**39.** 0.9

40. 4
41. 18
42. 16
43. 1350
44. 6
45. 36
46. 1 1/3
47. 8
48. 3.6
49. 450
50. 18
51. 657/1100, or 0.597
52. 3/5 or 0.6
53. 2 7/10
54. 2000
55. 171.43
56. 500
57. 10
58. 12 1/2 or 12.5
59. 240
60. 18 3/4
61. 6
62. 500
63. 62.4375
64. 180
65. 12 1/2
66. 80
67. 1/32, 0.03125
68. 100
69. 1620
70. 20

PROPORTIONS—POSTTEST 1, pp. 117-118

1. 2
2. 35/48
3. 6
4. 6.25
5. 32
6. 1/2
7. 2 1/2 or 2.5
8. 2
9. 5/9
10. 36
11. 4
12. 4
13. 8
14. 1500
15. 42
16. 4/9
17. 4
18. 100
19. 1
20. 3.2

PROPORTIONS—POSTTEST 2, pp. 119-120

1. 225
2. 1 7/25, 1.28
3. 120
4. 6.84
5. 13 1/3
6. 56
7. 1
8. 3.8
9. 3/20
10. 40
11. 3.6
12. 105
13. 2 7/10
14. 35/72
15. 10
16. 360
17. 15
18. 72
19. 1 2/25 or 1.08
20. 150

APOTHECARIES' AND HOUSEHOLD MEASUREMENTS—PRETEST, pp. 123-125

1. 1/3 ʒ
2. 6 ʒ, 3/4 ℥
3. 9 ℥, 4320 gr.
4. 4800 gr., 80 ʒ
5. 2 fl.ʒ, 1/4 fl. ℥
6. 5 fl.ʒ, 5/8 fl.℥
7. 1 9/16 fl.℥, 750 ♏
8. 20 fl.℥, 1 1/4 pt., 5/8 qt.
9. 96 fl.ʒ, 3/4 pt.
10. 512 fl.ʒ, 4 pt., 2 qt.
11. 80 fl.℥, 640 fl.ʒ, 2 1/2 qt.
12. 9600 ♏, 160 fl.ʒ, 20 fl.℥
13. 1 3/4 gal., 224 fl.℥
14. 640 fl.ʒ, 80 fl.℥, 5 pt.
15. 5 qt., 10 pt., 160 fl.℥
16. 24 fl.℥
17. 6 fl.ʒ
18. 10 ♏
19. 1 3/4 fl.ʒ
20. 15 fl.℥

APOTHECARIES' AND HOUSEHOLD MEASUREMENTS—WORK SHEET, pp. 131-134

Arabic to roman numerals, p. 131

1. xxii
2. ix
3. xliii
4. iii
5. clx
6. xviii
7. xxx
8. ccx
9. xiv
10. lxvii
11. xv
12. xxi
13. xii
14. xxvii
15. il

Roman to arabic numerals, p. 131

1. 29
2. 64
3. 7
4. 57
5. 104
6. 34
7. 6
8. 13
9. 19
10. 38
11. 40
12. 4
13. 25
14. 39
15. 240

Equivalents within apothecaries' system, pp. 131-133

1. 1/2 ʒ
2. 3 ʒ, 3/8 ℥
3. 1 13/24 ℥, 12 1/3 ʒ
4. 12 gr
5. 2 ℥, 960 gr
6. 65 ℥, 31,200 gr
7. 7 1/2 ℥, 3600 gr
8. 1 1/2 fl.ʒ, 3/16 fl.℥
9. 4 fl.ʒ, 1/2 fl.℥
10. 8 1/2 fl.ʒ, 1 1/16 fl.℥, 17/256 pt
11. 1/3 fl.ʒ
12. 1 1/2 fl. ℥
13. 1 1/4 fl.℥, 600 ♏
14. 2 1/2 fl.℥, 5/32 pt, 1200 ♏
15. 13/16 fl.℥, 390 ♏
16. 15 fl.℥, 15/16 pt, 15/32 qt
17. 8 fl.℥, 1/2 pt, 1/4 qt
18. 23,040 ♏, 384 fl.ʒ, 48 fl.℥
19. 512 fl.ʒ, 64 fl.℥, 2 qt
20. 40 fl.℥, 320 fl.ʒ, 19,200 ♏
21. 4 qt, 1 gal
22. 3840 ♏, 64 fl.ʒ, 8 fl.℥
23. 3/4 gal, 768 fl.ʒ, 6 pt
24. 20 pt, 320 fl.℥, 2 1/2 gal
25. 6 qt, 12 pt, 192 fl.℥

Household measures to equivalents in the apothecaries' system, pp. 133-134

26. 2 fl.ʒ
27. 4 fl.ʒ
28. 12 fl.ʒ, 1½ fl.℥
29. 10 fl.ʒ, 1¼ fl.℥
30. 10½ fl.℥, 84 fl.ʒ
31. 16 fl.℥
32. 10 ♏
33. 24 fl.ʒ, 3 fl.℥
34. 26 fl.℥, 208 fl.ʒ

APOTHECARIES' AND HOUSEHOLD MEASUREMENTS—POSTTEST 1, pp. 135-137

1. ¾ ʒ
2. 4 ʒ, ½ ℥
3. 45 ℥, 21,600 gr
4. 8½ ℥, 4080 gr
5. 1920 gr, 32 ʒ
6. 1⅔ fl.ʒ, 5/24 fl.℥
7. 5⅓ fl.ʒ, ⅔ fl.℥
8. 5 fl.℥, 2400 ♏, 5/16 pt
9. 22½ fl.℥, 1 13/32 pt, 45/64 qt
10. 80 fl.ʒ, ⅝ pt
11. 384 fl.ʒ, 3 pt, 1½ qt
12. 56 fl.℥, 448 fl.ʒ
13. 96 fl.ʒ, 12 fl.℥
14. 1¼ gal, 10 pt, 160 fl.℥, 1280 fl.ʒ
15. 7 qt, 14 pt, 224 fl.℥
16. 12 fl.℥
17. 4½ fl.℥
18. 12 fl.ʒ
19. 2½ fl.ʒ
20. 20 ♏

APOTHECARIES' AND HOUSEHOLD MEASUREMENTS—POSTTEST 2, pp. 139-141

1. ¼ ʒ
2. 5 ʒ, ⅝ ℥
3. 60 ℥, 28,800 gr
4. 2880 gr, 48 ʒ
5. 1⅚ fl.ʒ, 11/48 fl.℥
6. 5½ fl.ʒ, 11/16 fl.℥
7. 3¾ fl.℥, 1800 ♏, 15/64 pt
8. 26¼ fl.℥, 1 41/64 pt, 105/128 qt
9. 112 fl.ʒ, ⅞ pt
10. 576 fl.ʒ, 4½ pt, 2¼ qt
11. 72 fl.℥, 576 fl.ʒ
12. 1920 ♏, 32 fl.ʒ, 4 fl.℥
13. 1½ gal, 192 fl.℥
14. 832 fl.ʒ, 104 fl.℥, 6½ pt
15. 10 qt, 20 pt, 320 fl.℥
16. 20 fl.ʒ
17. 13½ fl.℥
18. 4 fl.℥
19. 3 fl.ʒ
20. 5 ♏

METRIC AND HOUSEHOLD MEASUREMENTS—PRETEST, pp. 143-145

1. 0.8 Gm
2. 3000 mcg
3. 0.255 Gm
4. 45 ml
5. 3 mg
6. 680 mg
7. 0.326 L
8. 72.6 lb
9. 2100 L
10. 3 kg
11. 100 ml
12. 10 ml
13. 5 cc
14. 800 Gm
15. 0.25 kl
16. 300 ml
17. 10,000 Gm
18. 630 ml
19. 0.733 kg
20. 1,250,000 mcg
21. 4 ml
22. 250 mcg
23. 600 L
24. 20.45 kg
25. 0.01 Gm
26. 1200 Gm
27. 300 ml
28. 710 mg
29. 0.48 L
30. 1 43/100 lb

METRIC AND HOUSEHOLD MEASUREMENTS—WORK SHEET, pp. 151-154

1. 0.00023 Gm
2. 5000 mcg
3. 2,500,000 mcg
4. 4 mg
5. 330 mg
6. 6000 Gm
7. 0.725 L
8. 0.002 Gm
9. 750 ml
10. 0.62 kg
11. 36 ml
12. 0.46 L
13. 660 mcg
14. 500,000 mcg
15. 0.474 kl
16. 0.35 Gm
17. 0.025 Gm
18. 1460 ml
19. 2500 Gm
20. 12,000 mcg
21. 3400 Gm
22. 0.00092 Gm
23. 0.25 kg
24. 0.3 mg
25. 160 ml
26. 10 mg
27. 5 mg
28. 0.36 Gm
29. 3,250 L
30. 450 mg
31. 0.24 L
32. 10 ml
33. 2 ml
34. 6 ml
35. 405 ml
36. 21 ml
37. 320 ml
38. 60 ml
39. 160 ml
40. 5 ml
41. 270 ml
42. 12 ml
43. 17⅗ lb
44. 8.415 lb
45. 4,318.18 Gm
46. 1.36 kg
47. 26⅖ lb
48. 3 2/25 lb
49. 10909.09 Gm
50. 68.18 kg

METRIC AND HOUSEHOLD MEASUREMENTS—POSTTEST 1, pp. 155-156

1. 0.005 Gm
2. 10,000 mcg
3. 810 ml
4. 0.035 Gm
5. 7 ml
6. 120,000 mcg
7. 35⅕ lb
8. 0.28 L
9. 400 Gm
10. 3 ml
11. 12727.27 Gm
12. 0.356 kg

13. 0.5 Gm
14. 0.037 L
15. 20 cc
16. 216 ml
17. 2500 mg
18. 12 ml
19. 6.7 kg
20. 300 L
21. 4000 mcg
22. $5\frac{18}{25}$ lb
23. 360 ml
24. 200 ml
25. 0.533 kl
26. 1,500,000 mcg
27. 0.62 Gm
28. 2500 Gm
29. 90 ml
30. 3.18 kg

METRIC AND HOUSEHOLD MEASUREMENTS—POSTTEST 2, pp. 157-158

1. 4 mg
2. 0.15 kg
3. 450 ml
4. $1\frac{19}{25}$ lb
5. $96\frac{4}{5}$ lb
6. 0.76 Gm
7. 550 ml
8. 0.788 kl
9. 80 ml
10. 965.909 Gm
11. 100 L
12. 32,000 mcg
13. 0.618 L
14. 0.1 Gm
15. 6 ml
16. 0.714 L
17. 0.35 kl
18. 0.25 Gm
19. 870 mg
20. 7000 mcg
21. 13 ml
22. 1400 L
23. 780 mg
24. 0.225 mg
25. 4.5 kg
26. 200 ml
27. 30 ml
28. 50 ml
29. 2,600,000 mcg
30. 33.18 kg

EQUIVALENTS—PRETEST, pp. 159-160

1. 12 ml
2. 28 ml
3. $79\frac{1}{5}$ lb
4. 5040 ml
5. 3 fl℥
6. 1.75 L
7. 6 Gm
8. $67\frac{1}{2}$ ♏
9. 3909.0909 Gm
10. 1080 ml
11. 210 ml
12. 0.6666 Gm
13. $5\frac{1}{2}$ qt
14. .3333 ml
15. 240 mg
16. 12 fl℥
17. $1\frac{1}{5}$ pt
18. $12\frac{1}{10}$ lb
19. 5 flʒ
20. $\frac{1}{5}$ gr
21. 0.2 mg
22. 38.6363 kg
23. $\frac{1}{150}$ gr
24. 36 ♏
25. $4\frac{1}{5}$ qt
26. 45 ml
27. 12 mg
28. 69 gr
29. 37.1° C
30. 105.8° F

EQUIVALENTS—WORK SHEET, pp. 165-168

1. $3\frac{1}{3}$ gr
2. 16 ml
3. 96 ml
4. 4 Gm
5. 75 flʒ
6. 10 Gm
7. 1750 ml
8. 7 fl℥
9. 2.6666 ml
10. 22 lb
11. $3\frac{1}{2}$ pt
12. 15 ml
13. 270 mg
14. $9\frac{6}{25}$ lb
15. 7 gr
16. 75 ♏
17. 3000 ml
18. $3\frac{1}{2}$ qt
19. 300 mg
20. 5 fl℥
21. 2 ml
22. 24 ml
23. $49\frac{1}{2}$ gr
24. 3090.909 Gm
25. 180 ♏
26. 12 ml
27. 165 mg
28. 105 gr
29. 2.2727 kg
30. $5\frac{2}{5}$ pt
31. 72 ml
32. $5\frac{2}{3}$ gr
33. 2.5 L
34. $8\frac{3}{100}$ lb
35. 6 qt
36. 32 ml
37. 120 ♏
38. 3 Gm
39. 3 ml
40. 120 ml
41. 5454.5454 Gm
42. $18\frac{3}{4}$ flʒ
43. 45 ♏
44. 34.0909 kg
45. 2125 ml
46. $1\frac{2}{3}$ gr
47. $3\frac{1}{2}$ qt
48. 90 mg
49. 1500 ml
50. 55 lb
51. 37.6° C
52. 38.8° C
53. 40.1° C
54. 36.3° C
55. 104.7° F
56. 95.7° F
57. 98.2° F
58. 102.6° F

EQUIVALENTS—POSTTEST 1, pp. 169-170

1. 180 mg
2. 0.8 ml
3. 20 ml
4. 5 Gm
5. 90 ml
6. 750 ml
7. $\frac{1}{4}$ gr
8. $1\frac{1}{2}$ qt
9. 3409.0909 Gm
10. 17.3333 ml
11. $1\frac{7}{10}$ qt
12. 0.3333 Gm
13. 2 flʒ
14. 9.0909 kg
15. 10 mg
16. 2 pt
17. 30 ♏
18. $\frac{1}{200}$ gr
19. 45 gr
20. 2 fl℥
21. $5\frac{47}{50}$ lb
22. 150 ml
23. $70\frac{2}{5}$ lb
24. $\frac{1}{120}$ gr
25. $22\frac{1}{2}$ ♏
26. 5.33 Gm
27. 2.75 L
28. 18 fl℥
29. 35.2° C
30. 96.1° F

EQUIVALENTS—POSTTEST 2, pp. 171-172

1. $64\frac{1}{2}$ ♏
2. 27.2727 kg
3. $2\frac{1}{2}$ qt
4. 0.2666 Gm
5. 625 ml
6. 15 mg

7. 1¼ qt
8. ⅓ gr
9. 1.5 ml
10. 9090.909 Gm
11. 375 ml
12. 2375 ml
13. 45 gr
14. 0.5 mg

15. 40 ml
16. 0.4666 Gm
17. 3.5 L
18. 3 pt
19. 2¹⁶⁄₂₅ lb
20. 0.6666 ml
21. ¹⁄₇₅ gr
22. 92⅖ lb

23. 48 ml
24. 3 mg
25. 21 ♏
26. 19½ gr
27. 1590.909 Gm
28. 2½ fl℥
29. 35.7° C
30. 100.8° F

ORAL DOSAGES—PRETEST, pp. 179-183

1. ½ tablet
2. 12 ml
3. 2 tablets
4. 1.33 ml
5. 15 ml
6. 2 tablets
7. ½ tablet

8. 2 tablets
9. 12.5 ml
10. 2 tablets
11. 8 ml
12. ½ tablet
13. 1½ tablet
14. 4 tablets

15. 1¹¹⁄₁₃ tablets (Give 2 tablets)
16. 2 capsules
17. 2 tablets
18. 15 ml
19. 2 capsules
20. 25 mg, 64 doses

ORAL DOSAGES—WORK SHEET, pp. 191-214

1. 2 capsules
2. 7.5 ml
3. 4 tablets, 3 tablets
4. 1 tablet
5. 2.5 ml
6. 24 doses
7. 2 capsules
8. 2 tablets
9. 4 ml
10. 2 tablets
11. 1 tablet
12. 2 tablets, 1200 mg
13. ½ tablet
14. ½ tablet
15. 1 tablet
16. 8 tablets, 4 tablets
17. 1.8 ml
18. ℥ 1, 120 ml
19. 12 ml
20. 4 tablets
21. 137.5 mg
22. 2 tablets
23. 2 capsules, 8 capsules
24. 15 ml ℥ 3¾
25. 7.5 ml
26. ½ tablet
27. 12 doses
28. ℥ 3
29. ½ tablet
30. 10 ml
31. ½ tablet
32. 3 tablets, 18 tablets
33. ℥ 2
34. 2 capsules
35. 25 ml
36. 60 ml
37. 3 tablets
38. 2 tablets, 600 mg
39. 9.38 ml
40. 2 tablets
41. 2 tablets
42. 2 tablets
43. 1 tablet
44. 2 tablets
45. 2 capsules, 8 capsules
46. ½ tablet
47. 3 tablets
48. 1.5 ml

49. 2 tablets
50. ℥ 2½
51. 4 capsules
52. 1 tablet
53. 2 capsules
54. 3 tsp
55. 3 tablets
56. 2 tablets
57. 3 ml
58. 6 capsules, 2 capsules, 8 capsules, 15 doses
59. 2.5 ml
60. 8.33 ml
61. 10 ml
62. ½ tablet
63. 3 tablets
64. 1.8 ml
65. 125 mg
66. 1 tablet
67. 3 capsules
68. ℥ 1, ℥ 8
69. 7.5 ml
70. ½ tablet
71. 2 tablets
72. 19.5 ml
73. 2 tablets
74. 50 mg
75. 3 ml
76. 2 tablets, 0.15 mg
77. 1½ tablets
78. 10 ml
79. 5 capsules
80. 20 mEq
81. ℥ 3⅔
82. 2 capsules
83. 1 tablet
84. 1 tablet, 200 mg, 600 mg
85. 2 tablets
86. 1200 mg
87. 2 capsules
88. 2 tablets
89. 1.33 ml
90. 6 mg
91. 2 capsules
92. ½ tablet
93. 4 tablets
94. 1 tablet
95. 2½ tablets
96. 6 ml

97. 3 tablets
98. 1 capsule
99. 30 ml
100. ½ tablet

ORAL DOSES—POSTTEST 1, pp. 215-219

1. 3 tablets
2. 1 capsule
3. 2 capsules
4. ʒ 4
5. 1 tablet
6. 12.5 ml
7. 2 tablets
8. 1 tablet
9. 2 tsp.
10. 0.5 Gm
11. ½ tablet
12. 15 ml
13. 4 tablets
14. 2 capsules
15. 0.9 ml
16. 4 ml
17. 250 mg
18. 2 tablets
19. 2 tablets
20. 1½ tablets, 4½ tablets

ORAL DOSAGES—POSTTEST 2, pp. 221-225

1. 2 capsules
2. 15 doses
3. 14.1 ♏
4. 3 tablets
5. 7.5 ml
6. 1 capsule
7. 3 tablets
8. 1 ml
9. 2 capsules
10. 1 7/65 tablet (give 1 tablet)
11. 9/10 tablet (give 1 tablet)
12. 10 ml
13. 4 tablets, 5 mg
14. 2 tablets
15. 100 mg
16. 1 4/5, (give 2 tablets)
17. 1 1/9, (give ʒ 1)
18. 3 tablets
19. 2 tablets
20. 3 tablets

PARENTERAL DOSAGES—PRETEST, pp. 227-231

1. 1 ml
2. 250 mg
3. 0.75 ml
4. 0.75 ml
5. 1 ml
6. 10 ♏
7. 2 ml
8. 2.2 ml
9. 8 ml
10. 0.5 ml
11. 0.58 ml
12. 0.4 ml
13. 2 2/5 ♏
14. 1 ml
15. 0.44 ml
16. 10 mg
17. 0.42 ml
18. 0.63 ml
19. 2 ml
20. 8 ml

PARENTERAL DOSAGES—WORK SHEET, pp. 239-260

1. 3 ml
2. 0.44 ml
3. 0.75 ml
4. 2 ml
5. 0.9 ml
6. 7.5 ml
7. 0.5 ml
8. 12 ml
9. 3 ml
10. 10 ♏
11. 28.9 ml
12. 4 ml
13. 30 ♏
14. 2.5 ml
15. 0.4 ml
16. 2.5 ml
17. 2 ml
18. 2 2/5 ♏
19. 0.25 ml
20. 0.25 ml
21. 0.5 ml
22. 15 ml
23. 2 ml
24. 0.5 ml
25. 1 ml
26. 18 ml
27. 0.8 ml
28. 2 ml
29. 0.4 ml
30. 2.22 ml
31. 2.5 ml
32. 0.8 ml
33. 3 ml
34. 150 mg
35. 1.5 ml
36. 1 ml
37. 1.5 ml
38. 3 ml
39. 1.5 ml
40. 3 ml
41. 0.5 ml
42. 1.6 ml
43. 0.5 ml
44. 3.6 ml
45. 1.07, (give 1 ml)
46. 20 ml
47. 0.5 ml
48. 0.8 ml
49. 10 ♏
50. 9 ♏
51. 30 mg
52. 3 ml
53. 1 ml
54. 3 9/20 ♏
55. 6.7 ml
56. 0.5 ml
57. 5 mg
58. 5 ml
59. 0.5 ml
60. 0.25 ml

61. 8 ml		**81.** 0.17 ml	
62. 0.5 ml		**82.** 1.6 ml	
63. 2 ml		**83.** 0.5 ml	
64. 1 ml		**84.** 15 m̃	
65. 0.7 ml		**85.** 5 mg	
66. 10.4 ml		**86.** 0.1 ml	
67. 0.3 ml		**87.** 1 ml	
68. 0.2 ml		**88.** 5.4 ml	
69. 1.375 ml, 1.38 ml		**89.** 18¾ m̃	
70. 0.3 ml		**90.** 0.6 ml	
71. 0.6 ml		**91.** 10 ml	
72. 1 ml		**92.** 2.25 ml	
73. 4 m̃		**93.** 0.4 ml	
74. 0.26 ml		**94.** 5 ml	
75. 1.4 ml		**95.** 1.6 ml	
76. 0.4 ml		**96.** 2 ml	
77. 6 ml		**97.** 1 ml	
78. 2 ml		**98.** 2 ml	
79. 2 ml		**99.** 0.2 ml	
80. 56¼ m̃		**100.** 0.4 ml	

PARENTERAL DOSAGES—POSTTEST 1, pp. 261-265

1. 2 ml		**11.** 1.4 ml	
2. 3³⁄₁₀ m̃		**12.** 0.5 ml	
3. 2 ml		**13.** 0.84 ml	
4. 5 ml		**14.** 2 ml	
5. 1 ml		**15.** 10 mg	
6. 0.25 ml		**16.** 0.6 ml	
7. 2 ml		**17.** 6 ml	
8. 0.5 ml		**18.** 1 ml	
9. 4 ml		**19.** 3 m̃	
10. 0.4 ml		**20.** 0.25 ml	

PARENTERAL DOSAGES—POSTTEST 2, pp. 267-271

1. 0.5 ml		**11.** 2 ml	
2. 0.5 ml		**12.** 20 m̃	
3. 8 ml		**13.** 5 ml	
4. 1.5 ml		**14.** 9¾ m̃	
5. 2 ml		**15.** 20 mg	
6. 0.3 ml		**16.** 4⅘ m̃	
7. 0.75 ml		**17.** 8 m̃	
8. 2.5 ml		**18.** 4 ml	
9. 1.375 ml (give 1.4 ml)		**19.** 1.67 ml	
10. 1.2 ml		**20.** 7.35 ml	

DOSAGES MEASURED IN UNITS—PRETEST, pp. 273-275

1. 0.5 ml	**5.** 5000 U
2. Insulin low-dose syringe with a vertical line at 16 U	**6.** 0.8 ml
3. 7.5 ml	**7.** Insulin low-dose syringe with vertical lines at 20 U and 25 U
4. 0.24 ml	**8.** 5⁷⁄₁₀ m̃

DOSAGES MEASURED IN UNITS—WORK SHEET, pp. 281-284

1. 2.5 ml	**9.** Insulin low-dose syringe with vertical lines at 14 U and 20 U
2. 1.5 ml	**10.** 3.75 ml
3. 3 m̃	**11.** 1.2 ml
4. 0.5 ml	**12.** Insulin low-dose syringe with a vertical line at 18 U
5. 0.5 ml	**13.** 0.32 ml
6. Insulin low-dose syringe with a vertical line at 2 U	**14.** 0.6 ml
7. 0.5 ml	**15.** 2 ml
8. 10 ml	

DOSAGES MEASURED IN UNITS—POSTTEST 1, pp. 285-287

1. 6.25 ml	**3.** 1.5 ml
2. 0.4 ml	**4.** Insulin low-dose syringe with a vertical line at 6 U

5. 3 ml

6. 0.4 ml

7. 2 ml

8. Insulin U-100 syringe with vertical lines at 38 U and 56 U

DOSAGES MEASURED IN UNITS—POSTTEST 2, pp. 289-291

1. Insulin low-dose syringe with a vertical line at 10 U

2. 1½ ℳ

3. 5 2½

4. 0.28 ml

5. 1.5 ml

6. 1.2 ml

7. 5¹⁄₁₀ ℳ

8. Insulin low-dose syringe with vertical lines at 16 U and 24 U

INTRAVENOUS FLOW RATES—PRETEST, pp. 293-295

1. 100 ml/h.	1.67 ml/min	25 gtt/min
2. 20.83 ml/h.	0.34 ml/min	20.83 gtt/min
3. 41.67 ml/h.	0.69 ml/min	8 gtt/min
4. 250 ml/h.	4.17 ml/min	42 gtt/min
5. 31.25 ml/h	0.52 ml/min	10 gtt/min

6. 0.2 U/ml, 10 ml/h, 0.17 ml/min, 10 gtt/min

7. 200 U/ml, 6 ml/h, 0.1 ml/min, 6 gtt/min

8. 825 μg, 4000 μg/ml, 0.20 ml/min, 12.37 gtt/min

INTRAVENOUS FLOW RATES—WORK SHEET, pp. 307-311

1. 125 ml/h.	2.08 ml/min	25 gtt/min
2. 100 ml/h.	1.67 ml/min	17 gtt/min
3. 125 ml/h.	2.08 ml/min	31 gtt/min
4. 150 ml/h.	2.5 ml/min	38 gtt/min
5. 62.5 ml/h.	1.04 ml/min	10 gtt/min
6. 100 ml/h.	1.67 ml/min	20 gtt/min
7. 125 ml/h.	2.08 ml/min	31 gtt/min
8. 93.75 ml/h.	1.56 ml/min	16 gtt/min
9. 10 ml/h.	0.17 ml/min	10 gtt/min
10. 83.33 ml/h.	1.39 ml/min	17 gtt/min
11. 133.33 ml/h.	2.22 ml/min	33 gtt/min
12. 2 ml/h.	0.03 ml/min	1.8 gtt/min

13. 0.4 U/ml, 30 ml/h, 0.5 ml/min, 30 gtt/min

14. 0.2 U/ml, 40 ml/h, 0.67 ml/min, 40 gtt/min

15. 20 U/ml, 5 ml/h, 0.08 ml/min, 5 gtt/min

16. 30 U/ml, 33.3 ml/h, 0.56 ml/min, 34 gtt/min

17. 900 μg/75 kg pt., 4000 μg/ml, 0.23 ml/min, 14 gtt/min

18. 22 mg/h/55 kg pt., 0.37 mg/min, 2 mg/ml, 0.19 ml/min, 11 gtt/min

19. 99 μg/min/66 kg pt., 200 μg/ml, 0.5 ml/min, 30 gtt/min

20. 400 μg, 1 mg (1000 μg)/ml, 0.4 ml/min, 24 gtt/min

INTRAVENOUS FLOW RATES—POSTTEST 1, pp. 313-314

1. 83.33 ml/h.	1.39 ml/min	21 gtt/min
2. 125 ml/h.	2.08 ml/min	25 gtt/min
3. 150 ml/h.	2.5 ml/min	38 gtt/min
4. 75 ml/h.	1.25 ml/min	13 gtt/min
5. 1.67 ml/min	20 gtt/min	

6. 0.5 U/ml, 8 ml/h, 0.3 ml/min, 18 gtt/min

7. 30 U/ml, 16.67 ml/h, 0.28 ml/min, 16.8 gtt/min

8. 246 μg/min/82 kg pt., 200 μg/ml, 1.23 ml/min, 73.8 gtt/min

INTRAVENOUS FLOW RATES—POSTTEST 2, pp. 315-316

1. 83.33 ml/h.	1.39 ml/min	21 gtt/min
2. 30 ml/h.	0.5 ml/min	10 gtt/min
3. 125 ml/h.	2.08 ml/min	25 gtt/min
4. 3 ml/h.	0.05 ml/min	3 gtt/min
5. 55.56 ml/h.	0.93 ml/min	9 gtt/min

6. 1 U/ml, 7 ml/h, 0.12 ml/min, 7 gtt/min

7. 30 U/ml, 50 ml/h, 0.83 ml/min, 50 gtt/min

8. 37.5 μg/min/75 kg pt., 20 μg/ml, 1.87 ml/min, 112.2 gtt/min

PEDIATRIC DOSAGES—PRETEST, pp. 317-318

1. 10.9 kg, 327-545 mg/day, yes, 0.05 ml

2. 10 kg, 60-75 mg/day, no

3. 40 kg, 5.6-80 mg/day, yes, 4 tablets
4. 23.6 kg, 23.6-52 mg/day, yes, 1 ml
5. 15.9 kg, 48-95 mg/day, yes, 1 ml

PEDIATRIC DOSAGES—WORK SHEET, pp. 321-323

1. 22.72 kg, 454.4-908.8 mg/day, yes, 1 capsule
2. 2.95 kg, 0.103-0.177 mg/day, no
3. 22.72 kg, 113.6 mg/day, yes, 0.4 ml
4. 20 kg, 11 mg/q 6 h., yes, 0.4 ml
5. 35.45 kg, 70.9 mg/day, yes, 1½ tablets
6. 13.77 kg, 27.54 mg/day, yes, 1 ml
7. 12.72 kg, 152.64 mg/day, yes, 1.42 ml
8. 30 kg, 150-210 mg/day, yes, 1½ tablets

PEDIATRIC DOSAGES—POSTTEST 1, pp. 325-326

1. 25 kg, 100-150 mg/day, yes, 15 ml
2. 20 kg, 600-1200 mg/day, no
3. 3 kg, 150,000 U/day, yes, 0.5 ml
4. 20 kg, 400-800 mg/day, yes, 10 ml
5. 35.45 kg, 3.54-7.09 mg/day, yes, 0.08 ml

PEDIATRIC DOSAGES—POSTTEST 2, pp. 327-328

1. 26.36 kg, 395-1054 mg/day, yes, 1.5 ml
2. 31.81 kg, 159-222.67 mg/day, no
3. 26.36 kg, 527-1054 mg/day, yes, 10 ml
4. 45 kg, 1125-2250 mg/day, yes, 2 capsules
5. 30 kg, 1500-3000 mg/day, yes, 4 ml

MATHEMATICS—PRETEST, pp. 341-346

1. A fraction whose numerator is larger than or equal to the denominator. ($36/4$)
2. A fraction whose numerator, denominator, or both contain fractions. ($\frac{1/3}{1/2}$)
3. The relationship between two numbers that are connected by a colon.
4. The number by which another number is divided. ($7\overline{)14}$)
5. A fraction consisting of a numerator that is expressed in numerals, a decimal point that designates the value of the denominator, and the denominator which is understood to be 10 or some power of 10.

6. $17/24$	**24.** 9	**42.** 0.0072	**59.** 42.3
7. $4\frac{2}{21}$	**25.** $8\frac{9}{40}$	**43.** 0.625	**60.** 292.5
8. $1\frac{16}{45}$	**26.** 27.413	**44.** 0.75	**61.** 3:14
9. $4\frac{9}{40}$	**27.** 1.827	**45.** 0.55	**62.** 9:16
10. 4.364	**28.** 31.79484	**46.** 0.68	**63.** 329:400
11. 33.832	**29.** 1579.2	**47.** $7/8$	**64.** 5:11
12. 13.058	**30.** $18/25$	**48.** $3/8$	**65.** 17:50
13. 34.659	**31.** $5/12$	**49.** $1/20$	**66.** 400
14. $1\frac{1}{12}$	**32.** $2/15$	**50.** $1/8$	**67.** 5
15. $23/30$	**33.** $33/80$	**51.** 43.2%	**68.** 24
16. $5/8$	**34.** 25.9924	**52.** $13/20$	**69.** $7\frac{1}{5}$ or 7.2
17. $1\frac{5}{6}$	**35.** 0.22625	**53.** 3:1000	**70.** 20
18. 1.053	**36.** 21.373	**54.** 12½% or 12.5%	**71.** 2000
19. 0.754	**37.** 6.4771	**55.** 20%	**72.** 100
20. 0.585	**38.** 0.003	**56.** 50%	**73.** 500
21. 1.417	**39.** 0.1	**57.** 7½% or 7.5%	**74.** 51
22. $1\frac{5}{7}$	**40.** 0.45	**58.** 0.15	**75.** 2½ or 2.5
23. $5/9$	**41.** 0.21		

9

reverse

① ml/hr   166 ml/hr

ml/min   166 : 1 min / x : 1 m   2.78 ml/hr

gtt/min   gttn
                drops / 1 ml : : gtt/min